# Praise for *Medical Answers Now!*

"The problems of American medical care are wide and deep. Dr. Burns, a thoughtful and committed primary care physician, has somehow found the time and energy to produce a compelling book packed with front-line experiences and a deep understanding of the plight of primary care in America. If we are to drag American healthcare out of the doldrums, it will require first saving Primary Care. Dr. Burns explains the role that Direct Primary Care will play in solving these problems. If you want to understand both the obstacles and solutions, I suggest that you read this book."

**Garrison Bliss, MD**, Internist and Founder of the Direct Primary Care movement

"Dr. Burns has written a revealing explanation of the underlying problems with our American healthcare system and outlines simple solutions for patients on how to get better access to affordable high-quality healthcare. Not only does this book clearly outline what you can do to always have access to your doctor when you need them but also will help you develop a fundamental understanding as to why the system is broken in the first place."

**Zak Holdsworth**, Co-founder & CEO, Hint Health

"Healthcare is in crisis around the globe, and in the United States. Confronted by burdens of ill health, limited resources, and confusing financial and healthcare systems, individuals and families often sense confusion, even desperation. Dr. Troy Burns illuminates these challenges and fluently describes solutions to healthcare that prove both physically effective and personally comforting."

**Nicholas Comninellis**, MD, MPH, Dean,
Institute for International Medicine

"While nobody can promise you a life without sickness or disease, Troy Burns, MD, reveals a simple path to significantly better health for about the price of your monthly cell phone bill. If you are a patient looking to improve your health or simply understand how to get better care, an employer trying to provide a better health benefit for your employees while hedging against the rising cost of care, or a policymaker trying to figure out how to make affordable primary care a reality for all—read this book today!"

**Jay Keese**, Executive Director,
Direct Primary Care Coalition

A DISRUPTIVE MODEL FOR HEALTHCARE
IN POST-PANDEMIC AMERICA

# MEDICAL ANSWERS NOW!

## HOW DIRECT PRIMARY CARE GUARANTEES FAST ACCESS TO YOUR DOCTOR

TROY A. BURNS, MD

*Medical Answers Now! How Direct Primary Care Guarantees Fast Access to Your Doctor*



**Medical disclaimer:** The information contained in this book is not intended as a substitute for the advice and/or medical care of the reader's physician, nor is it meant to discourage or dissuade the reader from seeking the advice of his or her physician. If the reader has any questions concerning the information presented in this book, or its application to his or her particular medical profile or the medical profile of a family member or friend, he or she should consult his or her physician. Neither the author nor the publisher shall be liable or responsible for any loss or damage allegedly arising as a consequence of the reader's use or application of any information or suggestions in this book. Patient privacy is respected under medical privacy laws.

This book reflects the individual views and opinions of Troy A. Burns, MD.

ISBN (paperback): 978-1-7379140-0-6
ISBN (ebook): 978-1-7379140-1-3
ISBN (audiobook): 978-1-7379140-2-0

Published by ProPartners Healthcare, P.A.
4501 College Blvd., #300
Leawood, KS 66211
www.propartnershealthcare.com
Contact the author: info@propartnershealthcare.com

To my wife, Cathy, six children, and two grandchildren (thus far). You have all taught me that the best qualities that a husband, father, and grandfather can aspire to are the same as those of a good physician and The Great Physician.

# Contents

Introduction ........ 1

Part I: You Need a Doctor ........ 5

1 Two Questions That Need Answers ........ 7

2 Scalpels and Pills: Illness and Injury ........ 21

3 The Long-Term Necessity of a Primary Care Relationship ........ 35

PART II: Why Is Getting the Medical Care I Need So Frustrating? ........ 49

4 The Current State of Primary Care in America ........ 51

5 Consequences of COVID-19 on Primary Care ........ 65

6 The Effects of Insurance Involvement on Primary Care ........ 79

PART III: How to Get Fast, Personal Care from Your Doctor ........ 93

7 The Triple Aim of Healthcare ........ 95

8 Value-Based Care and Direct Primary Care (DPC) ........ 109

9 How to Select and Establish Care with a Primary Care Physician ........ 125

10 Choosing Health Insurance to Complement DPC ...... 139

PART IV: Employee Health from the Care Up ........ 157

11 Direct Primary Care for Employers and Employees.... 159

12 Employer Selection of Medical Insurance to Complement DPC ........ 179

The Future of Healthcare: Next Steps to Improve Access to Care ........ 197

End Notes ........ 199

Acknowledgments ........ 223

About the Author ........ 227

# Introduction

More than 120 million Americans have been infected by the SARS-CoV-2 virus. Nearly two-thirds of our population has not been infected, but all of us have been affected. I am a primary care physician, and the majority of my time since March 2020 has been spent educating patients by aligning and applying guidance and mandates from healthcare and governmental authorities to the unique circumstances of individual patients.

The entire population has needed the support of trusted healthcare providers to help them make sense of the continuously evolving information related to disease mitigation, exposure, quarantine, isolation, symptoms, diagnostic approach, and treatments. These factors have brought to light not only the importance of high-level access to primary care but the current inadequacy of this access. People simply cannot get in to see a doctor.

While timely access to primary care has been proven to improve health and extend life, many people do not have a primary care physician, have neglected recommended care, and avoided seeing doctors to an even greater degree during the COVID-19 pandemic. In addition, access to primary care physicians has been even more restricted throughout the COVID-19 pandemic, and many patients are dissatisfied due to their inability to reach or be granted an appointment with their doctor in a timely manner. The typical/traditional insurance-participating primary care arrangements have also contributed to an environment that makes it very difficult for doctors to deliver quality care.

Here's what a new model of care looks like. And you can find these medical practices in your community. It's called Direct Primary Care or DPC. Since 2014, there has been a rapid nationwide expansion of physicians practicing in this new value-based primary care business model. DPC guarantees high-level access to your personal doctor and promises a savings in overall healthcare costs. You don't have to just imagine a world where you can see your doctor right away.

By the end of this book, you will have a firm understanding of these concepts so you can better manage your and your family's health:

- The value of having a personal primary care physician
- The current state of primary care in the US
- The triple aim of healthcare
- The effects of insurance involvement on the delivery of primary care
- The benefits of new value-based primary care models including DPC
- The six determining factors to look for in selecting your primary care physician

- How to identify and establish care with a new primary care physician
- How to select health insurance coverage to complement a Direct Primary Care arrangement with your personal physician

For business owners and decision-makers involved in employee benefits, you will see how DPC can form the foundation of health benefits and improve employee health and satisfaction with care while saving companies on overall healthcare costs.

The doctor will see you now.

# PART I

# YOU NEED A DOCTOR

# 1

# Two Questions That Need Answers

Sometimes you just want answers.

Google receives more than one billion health-related questions every day. That's an estimated 7% of all Google searches performed. Only a minority of these searches are for the purpose of finding a doctor. Most are people simply seeking health information and insight on their personal health, medical conditions, symptoms, medical test explanations, medications, nutrition, fitness, dietary supplements, or insurance questions.

Interestingly, health-related Google searches increase significantly in individuals who end up in the emergency room within the following two to three weeks. People clearly have health questions that require answers and often have pressing questions that, if not answered, may result in significant medical problems. As a practicing physician, I regularly see patients whose health outcomes would have been much better if they had been able to have their questions answered in a timely manner from a reliable and accurate source of information.

Jacqui, for example, knew something was wrong. Over the previous couple of weeks, she was having episodes of dizziness. Not just a little lightheadedness but actual spinning around vertigo. This was completely new to her so her instinct was to do her own research like she does for everything else in life—she Googled it. If only she knew what to believe.

She found a huge number of causes for vertigo and some were really scary. If she had one of those conditions, she needed to go to the ER right away. Then she remembered her doctor. She called our office, spoke with her physician on the phone, and was seen the same day. As it turns out, she didn't have a significant issue and was treated and reassured that her symptoms would likely resolve within another couple of weeks. Had she called sooner, she would not have had to worry and wonder what was wrong or what to do about it.

Contrary to popular belief, doctors really do appreciate it when their patients ask questions and take an active role in their own health. Asking questions and being engaged in the process of their own medical care is helpful to their doctor in delivering high-quality care, and it makes it much more likely that patients will comprehend and put into action the treatments and recommendations that their physician discusses with them. Even when patients' sources of information from an online health-related search are suspect or flat-out wrong, the inquiring mind absorbs much more of the accurate and necessary information that their physician (hopefully) shares and allows them to become true partners with their doctor in their ongoing health.

My son recently graduated from medical school, and I had the honor of "hooding" him (a proud dad moment when I draped the medical hood over his gown during the graduation ceremony). I felt like I should impart some kind of wisdom to help crystallize this new journey he was preparing to begin.

I told him that, in his entire career as a practicing physician in service to his patients, he will basically answer only two very important questions: *What's wrong with me?* and *What should I do about it?*

When people seek a doctor, they have a surprising breadth of questions, but the vast majority of them boil down to helping them understand the cause of their symptoms or health situation and then formulating a plan to address them. It seems simple, but it's surprising how often people seek answers from Dr. Google or even go to a physician's office and these fundamental questions go unanswered. These two questions need to be answered for everyone's health and peace of mind.

## What's Wrong with Me?

People want to know why.

The why is the *What's wrong with me?* question. It's the cause of their problem. The diagnosis. It's what doctors call the assessment. Not knowing what's going on in your body, if it is immediately dangerous or what it could mean for the future, understandably creates substantial anxiety and motivates people to seek an answer. Sometimes patients are much more worried about what it could be than they are in taking action to address it. They need an answer to this question—an answer that they trust, that relieves fear, and gives them confidence.

The *What's wrong with me?* questions are quite diverse. Have you ever asked yourself, a friend, Google, or your doctor any of these?

- I woke up with a runny nose and a cough. Do I have COVID?

- Why am I getting these chest pains? Am I having a heart attack?
- I have this dark mole on my leg. Is it skin cancer?
- Why can't I lose weight?
- My coworker tested positive for COVID. Now I don't feel good. Do I need to quarantine?
- I've been tired lately. Is it low testosterone?
- My back just keeps on hurting. Should I get an MRI? Do I have a herniated disk?
- Why does it take me so long to fall asleep?
- I've been getting these bad headaches lately that won't go away. Do I have a brain tumor?
- I get short of breath going up the stairs. Am I just out of shape or is there something else wrong with me?

The variety of questions that are brought to primary care physicians are much more varied than these. The questions often come from concern or fear more than they do the patient being affected by the severity of their symptoms. In many cases, patients are satisfied simply by knowing that they don't have something that is life-threatening or debilitating. They then return to their daily lives never feeling the need to take action to treat the actual symptoms.

So how do physicians go about accurately and completely answering a patient's burning question: *What's wrong with me?* We answer the question by asking questions. Asking and (ideally) listening carefully to our patients. Research over a span of more than thirty years has indicated that greater than 80% of the information a doctor needs to establish a diagnosis comes from asking the patient the right questions. Information gathered from taking the patient's history along with a focused and brief physical exam leads the doctor to what we call a differential diagnosis—a list of the most likely causes for the problem. Often this list is short or the diagnosis is completely obvious based on this information alone.

A minority of situations being presented to a doctor require the diagnosis to be established or confirmed by diagnostic tests like blood tests, imaging (x-ray, CT scans, MRIs), or other sophisticated diagnostic procedures. Of course, implicit in this process is that the doctor actually takes the time to ask those questions and obtain a thorough and accurate history of the patient's symptoms and situation. It takes time to ask and answer questions. As you may have experienced when visiting your doctor, this time allocation and attention to detail is far from guaranteed.

Getting the diagnosis or assessment correct is crucial to answering patients' inevitable second question: *What should I do about it?* If someone has a cough due to a cold, the treatment is obviously quite different than if their cough is caused by asthma, a sinus infection, acid reflux, or lung cancer. The doctor and the patient must have confidence in the accuracy of the assessment in order to pursue an appropriate and effective treatment. You need a doctor to answer both questions.

## What Should I Do about It?

People want to know what they should do about a health issue.

In some cases, patients will go to their doctor already knowing or suspecting the cause of their concern. In most cases, the doctor will help them figure it out. In either case, when the patient is confident that they have the answer to the question, *What's wrong with me?* they logically want an answer to the follow-up question, *What should I do about it?*

After diagnosis comes treatment, or in doctor terms, after assessment comes a plan. A medically advised plan may include prescription or over-the-counter medications or lifestyle modifications such as quitting smoking, cutting back on alcohol, improving diet, increasing exercise, or losing weight. The plan may also include surgeries, allied health therapies, vaccinations, and an array of other treatment procedures. There are typically also recommendations for follow-up, which may include additional tests or repeat examination to observe and document progress toward returning to a normal or healthier state.

The *What should I do about it?* questions, after a diagnosis is established, are also quite varied. These examples provide a sense of the range of the questions about recommendations or treatment that need to be answered.

- So my COVID test was positive? Now what? Should I isolate at home? Can you prescribe ivermectin? Hydroxychloroquine? What else should I do?
- How can I keep myself from getting skin cancer?
- What is the best diet to help me lose weight?
- So I did have a heart attack. Do I need bypass surgery? How can I keep this from happening again?
- I've heard testosterone will really help guys my age. Will you prescribe testosterone for me?

- The MRI shows a herniated disk. Do I need surgery? What else can we do?
- My wife says I stop breathing during the night. Should I get one of those CPAP things?
- I'm really feeling stressed a lot and I don't know what to do. It's really getting to me. What should I do?

As with investigating a patient's health concerns and establishing an assessment or diagnosis, the doctor must use all of their training, experience, and expertise to develop an effective plan of action. However, the best laid plans for treatment that fully answer the question *What should I do about it?* are meaningless if they aren't agreed upon by the patient and then put into action. It has been well established that compliance with medical treatment recommendations is directly related to how well the patient understands their doctor's recommendations and the rationale for them.

Ample time with the doctor discussing the why of their recommendations and treatments makes it considerably more likely that patients will comply and achieve favorable outcomes. Patient compliance is based on understanding. Again, it takes time.

Ultimately, doctors answer two questions. And they give advice. In my practice, I learned long ago that, just as I am unable to make my adult children do what I think they should, I cannot make any patient follow my advice, no matter how wonderful, important, or life-saving that I think it is. It's just advice. It is the patient's responsibility to take the doctor's advice—or leave it. The best doctors build trust, involve their patients in decision-making, and become partners with patients in final treatment decisions.

The question *What should I do about it?* is most appropriately, *What should **we** do about it?* as proactive partners in your health. This is the reason my medical practice is named ProPartners Healthcare! This approach and honest perspective, especially from a primary care physician, improves patient care, satisfaction with care, and health outcomes. Patients benefit from the answers to their two questions only if they understand and trust their doctor. You need a doctor that you trust.

## Trusted Advice and Information

Getting answers to two questions isn't really the whole story.

People want answers. But they want good answers, answers that they trust, from sources that they trust within a primary healthcare relationship that they trust with a doctor who knows them.

Technology has put nearly infinite amounts of information on every subject in the palm of our hand. We have the ability to get answers to all of our questions almost immediately wherever we are. Ask Siri and Google returns multiple "answers" to the one billion health-related questions they receive every day. Some of those answers are accurate and trustworthy. But which ones?

In the advertising world, they say half of all advertisements work, they just don't know which half. In internet searches for health information, people have the same problem. There are so many sources of information. Most searches return results that largely consist of the unsubstantiated opinions of writers, promotional pitches of people and companies trying to sell products, or anecdotal arguments and advice. At best, a search gives a conflicting, contradictory, and obviously confusing picture on nearly every medical topic, especially to the majority of people without a medical background. At worst, following the wrong advice is truly dangerous.

"Don't believe everything you read" used to be common knowledge. In seeking health information, as in life, this idiom is a much-needed warning to us all. Not only must we not believe everything we read and hear, but it may be dangerous to believe everything that we think.

How often have you firmly believed something that turned out to be wrong? Have you ever watched the TV news or read a newspaper? Overconfidence in our own interpretation of information that we have cobbled together in an area that is not our expertise can get us into trouble, especially when it comes to our health. So what and whom should you believe? Who can you trust when it comes to your health?

As you might have figured out, this book is ultimately about finding your single primary source of health information and peace of mind about your medical care in a relationship with a highly accessible primary care physician. You need this kind of doctor.

In a long-term trusting relationship with a physician who knows you, health questions expand from the immediate *What's wrong with me?* and *What should I do about it?* into broader questions and discussions with your doctor about general health, preventive care, and quality of life. Of course, it is ideal when doctors have the opportunity to advise their patients about health-related matters before they develop medical conditions. This is the beginning of effective preventive care. When primary care physicians prioritize this role, they discuss and answer important questions like these:

- I read that I should check my cortisol level because I don't have the energy I used to and I might have inflammation or a problem with my adrenal gland. What do you think, Doc?
- Can I send you this article I read about intermittent fasting? I want to get your opinion.
- I'm really struggling. I just found out my husband is having an affair and I just don't know what to do. I'm not eating or sleeping. What should I do?
- I heard this ad on the radio for low T. Is this something I should look into?
- My wife and her friends are all taking bee pollen to help them lose weight and are convinced it is really helping them. Is there something to this? Should I take it?
- I'm not an alcoholic but sometimes feel like I should drink less. Am I hurting myself drinking a couple of drinks after dinner?
- I saw a commercial for a new drug for my psoriasis. Should I try it?

SARS-CoV-2 (the virus that caused the COVID-19 pandemic) proved to be a perfect example of people's desire and need for a trusted medical adviser. As a primary care physician in a medical practice that allows patients direct access to their doctor via phone and text, I spent the majority of my time during the pandemic discussing patients' situations and their questions related to exposures, symptoms, and concerns about COVID-19. Throughout the pandemic, information from health authorities and politicians was constantly changing, evolving, conflicting, and creating confusion. People learned what scientists have always known, that "following the science," by definition, means wandering in the desert while research proves or disproves various hypotheses.

My patients like everyone else were just looking for clear advice from someone they trusted to know the current state of knowledge about the virus and the pandemic. They wanted me to put information, as we knew it at the time, into context and reasonably apply the guidance of the CDC and state and local health authorities as well as keeping them up-to-date on state and local mandates that had been in place.

Peace of mind! The desired effect of answers to your health questions from a source that you trust brings peace of mind. Primary care physicians provide a single source for their patients on a wide range of health conditions and subjects in the context of a long-term relationship. Peace of mind comes when that trusted source is someone you know, someone who has a breadth of health information, who can translate from technical language, and who gives you a way to put all of that information into context.

## From My Practice

Bill, age forty-three, had been a patient of mine for about nine years. He was generally healthy but admitted to drinking a little too much on the weekends and overdoing it with unhealthy and spicy food. He had put on the COVID twenty (pounds) through the pandemic and started to have frequent heartburn along with the feeling that food was getting stuck in his throat when he swallowed certain kinds of foods over the previous month. By the time he came to see me, he was eating TUMS like candy and was wondering if he had an ulcer. He had the two questions: *What's wrong with me?* (an ulcer?) and *What should I do about it?* He wanted and needed answers now.

My job was to first answer his *What's wrong with me?* question by making a diagnosis. By asking Bill several questions and performing a brief exam, I concluded that his issue was with his esophagus and/or his stomach. The possibilities (differential diagnosis) included reflux esophagitis (GERD), an esophageal stricture/narrowing, an ulcer (peptic ulcer disease), or something worse like an esophageal or stomach cancer. Fortunately, I could give him some reassurance that his condition was more likely to be something that was not life-threatening, was not highly likely to be an ulcer or stomach cancer, and could be quickly and effectively treated. That delivered the peace of mind that he was looking for.

Next, Bill needed to know *What should I do about it?* We discussed the options for initial treatment and agreed on trying a prescription stomach acid medication (proton pump inhibitor) for a couple of weeks. I further explained that if all his symptoms resolved (went away) completely, we had our likely diagnosis, and he would not require any additional tests or treatments. If the symptoms did not go away, he would need to see a specialist in gastroenterology who would probably recommend an upper endoscopy (EGD) to rule out esophageal stricture, ulcer, and cancer.

As it turns out, his symptoms did not fully resolve; I referred him to a gastroenterologist who performed a scope, which ruled out those more concerning diagnoses. His symptoms eventually resolved on the medication I had initially prescribed. Bill made a point to circle back to express his gratefulness to me for figuring out what was wrong with him and what he should do about it in a way that gave him information, perspective, and context, allayed his fears, and reassured him that he was in good hands.

## What Do We Know?

Just like Bill, you need a doctor. You need a doctor because you have health questions that need to be answered. You have the two fundamental questions *What's wrong with me?* and *What should I do about it?* that come up again and again in endless variations. Since information is plentiful but accurate information is elusive and clarity is scarce, you want answers from someone who knows you, someone that you trust to make sense of your situation (assessment), and someone who can give you good advice (recommendations) about what to do about it.

Primary care physicians exist to provide you with these answers. As it turns out, not only do you need these answers, but sometimes you need them now.

# 2

# Scalpels and Pills: Illness and Injury

Sometimes, as a patient, you need answers NOW!

People have all kinds of health questions. Some are mere curiosity. Some are general questions about their long-term health. Some relate to nagging symptoms they have had for a long time, but some concerns aren't so casual, really can't wait, and require treatment right away.

When you have a pressing medical need, what do you do? Maybe you feel sick, have pain, or just got injured. You need attention immediately. Right now. Acute illnesses and injuries can't wait. In addition to providing information, a main function of a primary care physician is to provide treatment in a timely manner. You know you need to see a doctor right away. You could just go to the emergency room or an urgent care walk-in clinic, but you wish you could see a doctor that you know and trust—a doctor who knows you. If you could get your doctor on the phone or see them in the office today, you know that would be best.

Just as doctors primarily answer the two vital questions discussed in the first chapter when making recommendations to patients (*What's wrong with me?* and *What should I do about it?*), when it comes to treating them, we also typically do two things: we cut on you or give you pills. Sure, we sometimes tell you what to eat, to get more exercise or lose weight, but for the most part the treatments prescribed by physicians usually boil down to either prescribing medications or performing a surgical procedure.

When you are on your smartphone, no matter what you want to do, there's an app for that. If you go to the doctor, there's always a pill for that. Modern medicine has advanced remarkably in our lifetime with the development of complex and precise surgical procedures and prescription medications that treat trauma, chronic diseases, and acute conditions more effectively than anyone would have imagined a few decades ago.

When these "scalpels and pills" are put to work quickly, they routinely save lives. And while this description is a simple reduction of a broad range of medical treatments, starting the appropriate treatment as soon as possible often determines the outcome. The sooner a treatment is begun, the more likely and more quickly you, the patient, are to fully recover.

For most illnesses, escalating medical problems, and acute injuries, when you decide that you need to see a doctor, you want to do it now, not tomorrow or next week. How fast you can get in front of a doctor who can diagnose and treat you makes all the difference. Timely access to your primary care physician usually determines the quality of your care, how quickly you initiate treatment, and consequently how quickly you recover.

## Injury

A major category of medical need that requires answers and treatment now is injuries.

According to the CDC, there are approximately 35 million injury-related visits to US emergency departments each year. That's 27% of all ER visits. While many of these injuries may have been best managed in other settings such as primary care offices or urgent care walk-in clinics, the most severe and obvious traumas are handled at hospital-based emergency departments.

If you have a true traumatic injury that immediately debilitates you or that you or others around you believe could be life-threatening (let's say a broken leg or hip or you're unconscious from a fall or something involving loss of blood), you are calling an ambulance or being taken to the ER. This is the most obvious situation that requires true emergency care immediately and is more likely to require a surgical treatment or hospitalization.

Fortunately, in most of the US everyone will be treated emergently at highly qualified trauma centers without regard to insurance or ability to pay. Treatment now happens reliably in these circumstances and occurs in the only appropriate setting.

Unfortunately, many of the 35 million ER visits for injuries do not require the high-level trauma and emergency services that are available at a hospital emergency department and therefore result in many unnecessary and expensive trips to the ER. The most common unnecessary ER visits are for pain. The vast majority of people with headaches, back pain, toothaches, and sore throats should find a better and more cost-effective way to get help. A portion of these unnecessary ER visits seemed necessary to individuals because they could not reach their personal physician or their doctor could not accommodate them into their schedule immediately or on the same day. They simply did not know where else to go for timely care.

Most acute injuries do not require care at the emergency department of a hospital but often need to be addressed by a doctor on the same day that they occur. Each year in the US there are an additional 39.5 million doctors' office visits for injuries. Acute injuries like sprains, strains, lacerations, abrasions, bruises, many broken bones, concussions and other injuries from falls, collisions, bicycle accidents, equipment injuries, and more may be serious and require urgent treatment by a doctor but are handled more efficiently and cost-effectively in the ambulatory care setting of a doctor's office or urgent care clinic.

As I will highlight in future chapters of this book, primary care physicians are fully trained and ideally suited to treat these injuries in their offices. Primary care physicians assess and initiate treatment of these injuries, order diagnostic tests such as x-rays or other imaging studies, and arrange for same-day referrals to specialists if they are needed.

I find that many of my patients are surprised that primary care physicians have years of experience with sewing up lacerations, applying splints and casts, and dealing with other injuries that they assumed would require an ER visit or a specialist. Initial injury care by primary care physicians saves many injured people a lot of wasted time and money at the ER and also often saves employers on health insurance claims and healthcare costs in general.

But what about those less acute, ongoing, or nagging injuries that you have tried to handle on your own and just hoped they would go away over time? They may have been lingering, not getting better for weeks or months but are getting worse to the degree that you can't stand it another day. There are a million examples of prolonged symptoms from these types of subacute injuries: that kink in your neck, chronic low back pain, tendinitis in your elbow or shoulder, swollen knee, or pain in your big toe. As we get older, the list of nagging pains or injuries that aren't necessarily getting worse but aren't going away can go on and on.

When you finally decide you need help, you want it now. Where do you go for help with these kinds of problems? Do you need an orthopedist or a rheumatologist? With these types of ongoing injuries, you would also ideally get answers, advice, and treatment from the doctor who knows you best: your primary care physician—if they could see you right away.

## Illness

Injuries aren't the only pressing medical needs that require medical care right away.

Just as some injuries are immediately life-threatening and must be handled at the hospital emergency department, some medical conditions and symptoms of illness are also true medical emergencies. These conditions can cause disability or death and must be taken seriously as soon as they develop. It is important to know the kinds of symptoms that are red flags for serious or life-threatening emergencies.

If you ever develop any of these serious symptoms, they must be evaluated and treated as soon as possible since the time from onset of symptoms until treatment is initiated greatly determines your outcome and may even save your life. According to the American College of Emergency Physicians, the following symptoms represent medical emergencies that require help right away:

- Bleeding that will not stop
- Breathing problems (difficulty breathing, shortness of breath)
- Change in mental status (such as unusual behavior, confusion, difficulty arousing)
- Chest pain
- Choking
- Coughing up or vomiting blood
- Fainting or loss of consciousness
- Feeling of committing suicide or murder
- Severe or persistent vomiting
- Sudden, severe pain anywhere in the body
- Sudden dizziness, weakness, or change in vision
- Swallowing a poisonous substance
- Severe abdominal pain or pressure

If any of these symptoms are present to a significant degree, your best bet is to have someone take you to the hospital ER immediately. If you aren't sure the symptoms are significant enough to warrant a trip to the ER and you can reach your doctor right away, you may be able to get professional advice as to whether you need to go to the ER. If you can't, you essentially have no choice but to head to the hospital ER. In these situations, you will obviously benefit from initial answers to those two universal questions: *What's wrong with me?* and *What should I do about it?*

Most illnesses and symptoms not on the previous list do not require assessment and treatment at the hospital emergency department, but that doesn't mean that their evaluation and treatment can or should be put off to another day. Most acute illnesses or symptoms do not warrant expensive emergency care but are best handled quickly. You really may need answers and help now.

Certain infections and medical conditions such as the flu, sinus infections, ear infections, strep throat, pneumonia, acid reflux, stomach ulcers, vomiting and diarrhea, diverticulitis, diabetes, high blood pressure, urinary infections, gout, and countless others should be treated right away. These conditions can typically be diagnosed quickly by a doctor and then cured or brought under control in short order. As in the case of injuries, the timely care of illnesses and medical symptoms is essential to your recovery and ongoing health.

Just as with chronic nagging injuries, most people tolerate chronic nagging medical symptoms for some period of time until it's obvious that they aren't going away or are actually getting worse. Patients are equally likely to be chastised by doctors for waiting too long before seeking medical care as they are for coming to the doctor too quickly after a symptom starts. Sometimes nagging symptoms represent illnesses or infections that are quickly cured and gone, but they may, in some cases, be indicators of chronic diseases or life-threatening medical conditions.

Patients frequently come to my office with vague symptoms that turn out to be untreated diabetes, cardiovascular disease, neurologic problems, thyroid disease, inflammatory bowel disease, any number of types of cancer, or a myriad of other medical problems that will require lifelong management. If you could only get your doctor on the phone to ask if your symptoms warrant a trip to their office. You need a doctor.

## Treatment Now (from a Doctor You Know)

People often need to be treated immediately. But they understandably prefer to see someone that they know—a doctor who knows them and has a proven track record of helping them through illnesses and injuries in the past. A physician with whom they already have a well-established relationship.

If you are in the midst of a life-threatening injury or medical condition, you're not going to be interviewing the doctor or insisting to see someone that you know. In all other circumstances, you will feel more comfortable and confident if you can receive information and care from a doctor who already knows you and your medical history. You have common history, have trusted them with other medical problems, and they have proven themselves to be of value to you. You intuitively know what is common knowledge in the medical community: it is much easier for a physician to provide high-quality medical care to someone whose medical history and personal history is already well known to them.

As a primary care physician, my job is made much easier by having a context in which to diagnose and treat each of my patients. One of the first orders of business, preferably soon after meeting a new patient, is to schedule a comprehensive preventive health assessment or check-up. During this visit, I will review my new patient's current medications, allergies to medications or food, immunizations, currently treated medical conditions, history of surgeries and hospitalizations, past medical and psychological problems, family history, social history (relationships, children, occupation, for example), history of tobacco use, alcohol, caffeine, illicit drugs, dietary and exercise habits, inquire about a long list of symptoms that patients may have and also ask about any other physicians that the patient sees regularly.

In addition, I invite each patient to share any health concerns they may have during the visit that didn't come up during our comprehensive history-taking process. Finally, I will perform a general head-to-toe physical examination, measure height and weight, take vital signs, and obtain a broad panel of baseline blood tests.

This thorough initial assessment gives me indispensable information and a clear advantage in accurately diagnosing and treating my patients in the future. There is simply no way that a random doctor in an urgent care clinic, emergency room, or on the other end of a telemedicine phone call can know my patients the way that I do or will be able to treat them with as much insight as I can, just because I have gone through this process.

As important as all of this baseline medical information is to ongoing care, another aspect of primary care is arguably more important. It is relationship. Over time, primary care physicians have the opportunity to really get to know their patients. In addition to the medical care we provide with as much empathy as we know how, we are also often with them through their challenges with work and family. We provide a listening ear and encouragement (in addition to pills) through difficult times in their lives including marital problems, divorces, behavior problems with children, job losses, and deaths of their family members and close friends.

These shared experiences and assistance are indispensable to truly understanding our patients and knowing how to communicate and explain things to them in a way that is unique to each patient, that they will understand and will benefit them personally.

Over the years of a long-standing doctor-patient relationship, patients gain the most valuable benefit they can have in any relationship: trust. As it relates to this working relationship with your personal physician, trust leads to confidence and confidence gives peace of mind. In the context of repeated encounters with your doctor, your confidence builds in their ability to reliably answer the questions *What's wrong with me?* and *What can I do about it?* And your confidence in their treatment recommendations, whether they be medications, surgical procedures, lifestyle modifications, or referrals to specialized physicians, should continue to grow and give you peace of mind even when faced with difficult medical situations.

Repeatedly seeking medical treatment first from a doctor that you know well also conveys the benefit of what medical professionals call continuity of care. The American Academy of Family Physicians defines continuity of care:

> Continuity of care is concerned with quality of care over time. It is the process by which the patient and his/her physician-led care team are cooperatively involved in ongoing health care management toward the shared goal of high-quality, cost-effective medical care. Continuity of care is a hallmark and primary objective of family medicine and is consistent with quality patient care provided through a medical home. The continuity of care inherent in family medicine helps family

physicians gain their patients' confidence and enables family physicians to be more effective patient advocates. It also facilitates the family physician's role as a cost-effective coordinator of the patient's health services by making early recognition of problems possible. Continuity of care is rooted in a long-term patient-physician partnership in which the physician knows the patient's history from experience and can integrate new information and decisions from a whole-person perspective efficiently without extensive investigation or record review.

## From My Practice

I was mowing my lawn on a sunny Saturday morning in suburban Kansas City and received a text from one of my patients (yes, my patients can text me directly on my personal mobile phone) who had just sliced his thumb with a box knife. John, at age fifty-nine, had been a patient of mine for about fourteen years. It was obvious to him that he needed stitches and a tetanus shot. In this case, he didn't need an answer to the question *What's wrong with me?* He was just asking his doctor what he should do about it. He needed help now.

As you might guess, John assumed that I would tell him to go to the hospital emergency department (where he would write a big check) or to an area urgent care since our offices are closed on the weekend. Because I was available and my office wasn't too far from either of us, I was willing to open the office and help him out. I knew he would prefer to have his personal physician take care of him and that I could save him as much money by avoiding the ER as he would pay me for all of my services in the coming year or more.

I told him I would finish mowing and then meet him at my office to take care of him. We both arrived at my office about an hour later. His care would have been simple for any primary care physician (even though my office staff wasn't there to help). I set up the surgical tray and instruments, drew up the anesthetic, donned my sterile gloves, cleaned up his wound, and put in a few stitches. After I figured out where my staff kept the tetanus vaccine, I drew that up and gave it to him as well. The whole visit took only about fifteen minutes, and John was happily on his way (albeit with a sore thumb and instructions on how to watch for infection).

Only because John could reach his personal physician by phone (text) immediately and I was willing to take care of him right away, his medical care, patient experience (satisfaction), and cost of care was far better than it would have been if he had not been in a primary care relationship with a physician whose practice is designed for high-level access and availability. He needed treatment now. He preferred and was able to receive that care from his personal physician whom he trusts and who knows him well.

## It's All about Access

Sooner or later, you will need answers about your health without waiting, and you will need medical treatment on the same day a health issue arises. You need a doctor.

Whether you've thought of it or not, you want and need answers now! Answers for information. Answers now and treatment now for illnesses and injuries. You may need pills. You may need a scalpel or other minor procedure. You may simply need guidance or advice, but you really will need it now. If you've ever been frustrated (or always been frustrated) when you have an immediate need for a doctor, please read on. You really can guarantee timely access to a personal primary care doctor whenever you need it.

Even more important than many urgent interventions for illnesses and injuries is the broader long-term value of preventive care that can improve the quality and duration of your life. This may even be the most important reason that you need a doctor. Health education and counseling, preventive care, timely screening for disease, and encouragement to pursue a healthy lifestyle are the most beneficial when they are delivered in the context of a supportive long-term relationship with a primary care physician who knows you well and that you trust to give you answers and advice about your health.

# 3

# The Long-Term Necessity of a Primary Care Relationship

You need a doctor for more than just urgent medical questions and treatments. Take Malia, for example. She was a typical teen who struggled with her self-esteem and also with her weight. It wasn't an urgent medical problem, but it was always on her mind and affected her happiness, her relationships, and her success. She had never really brought up her concerns with anyone. Not her friends or her parents.

Fortunately, when in a "well-child" check-up at our office, she worked up the nerve to write it on one of the office's medical history questionnaires that is confidential, just between Malia and her doctor. She trusted her doctor (my partner) enough to confide in her and begin to address this very important issue.

Like Malia, you (and every patient) want to receive answers now from a doctor that you know and trust. That doctor-patient relationship is crucially important. You should recognize that the value of having a primary care physician extends well beyond securing quick access for life's unexpected emergencies.

In this chapter I discuss a full and functional definition of the breadth of primary care services as well as the five primary benefits that having a long-term relationship with a personal primary care physician offers you. These benefits include the broad scope of issues that primary care physicians address:

- Continuity and accountability of care
- Proactive preventive care
- Assistance in navigating the overall healthcare system
- Ultimately better health with lower healthcare costs

You will see that these benefits are crucial to lifelong health and longevity, and they also improve patient satisfaction with medical services while providing increased efficiency and more cost-effective care.

## What Is Primary Care?

Americans receive medical care in many ways.

Too often in the United States, the delivery of healthcare is done in a manner that is piecemeal, inefficient, and unnecessarily expensive. It is not uncommon for people to receive initial care from multiple providers in disparate medical practice settings and institutions. They may go to urgent care walk-in clinics as their primary first stop for illnesses and emergency departments at hospitals for even minor injuries. In addition, they may see a cardiologist for their high blood pressure, an endocrinologist for simple type 2 diabetes, an allergist for seasonal allergies, and an orthopedist for chronic knee pain. It is also increasingly common for people to utilize some kind of telemedicine service, which puts them on the phone or a video call with a physician they have never met to address an acute medical concern.

In this example alone, a patient without a primary care physician may be seeing seven different physicians and medical groups for very common and routine conditions. As you might imagine, this widely dispersed care is inefficient, costly, and creates a situation that makes it nearly impossible for providers to smoothly coordinate the patient's care.

There is a better way—a first stop for all medical questions and needs. A medical home where the majority of medical concerns are diagnosed and treated by a single physician and where any specialty care that is required is coordinated on behalf of the patient. Primary care physicians or PCPs are the doctors who fulfill this role for their patients. They are most often trained in family medicine, internal medicine, pediatrics, or general practice and are well-equipped to handle the majority of health issues that patients may have. They are also alert to triage or refer their patients to any number of other physician specialists when needs arise. Not surprisingly, common things occur commonly. Primary care physicians "specialize" in common conditions and health needs.

A discussion of the value of primary healthcare must begin with a definition of the practice. A functional definition is found in a text by Cruz-Cunha and associates:

> Primary care involves the widest scope of healthcare, including all ages of patients, patients of all socioeconomic and geographic origins, patients seeking to maintain optimal health, and patients with

> all manner of acute and chronic physical, mental and social health issues, including multiple chronic diseases. Consequently, a primary care practitioner must possess a wide breadth of knowledge in many areas. Continuity is a key characteristic of primary care, as patients usually prefer to consult the same practitioner for routine check-ups and preventive care, health education, and every time they require an initial consultation about a new health problem. Collaboration among providers is a desirable characteristic of primary care.

Primary care is generally accepted to be the foundation of any effective healthcare system. Effective and efficient healthcare begins with a single primary physician who has an ongoing relationship with the patient, a detailed knowledge of their medical and personal history over time, and is trusted by the patient to be the first source of information, advice, diagnosis, and treatment of their health needs. In the context of this relationship, patients are statistically more likely to receive timely preventive screenings, early detection and treatment of diseases, and well-balanced health education and are more likely to be encouraged in lifestyle modification and healthy lifestyle. Primary care improves health, prevents illness and death, and is also associated with a more equitable distribution of health in populations.

During the COVID-19 pandemic, individuals with primary care relationships were better able to receive appropriate medical care, diagnosis, and treatment of COVID-19 infection and had a medical consultant to explain confusing mitigation guidance and mandates as questions arose. Primary care physicians also serve as a medical home for their patients, referring and coordinating consultations of specialists and explaining/interpreting the recommendations of these specialists to their patients.

## Five Benefits of a Primary Care Relationship

Medical doctors practicing as primary care physicians (PCPs) are the only physicians who deliver all of the following five major benefits of a primary care relationship to their patients. All five of these aspects of care are required for any person to receive well-coordinated overall medical and preventive care with a high level of continuity of care in the most efficient and cost-effective manner possible.

What are these five benefits and why are they necessary for the best quality healthcare?

### *1. Address the Vast Majority of Healthcare Needs*

Primary care physicians are able to address and solely manage the vast majority of healthcare needs. In a study in *JAMA Internal Medicine* (2012), researchers estimated that more than 90% of concerns that are brought to primary care doctors are successfully dealt with without the need for referral to any specialist physician. Due to the broad training and scope of practice of primary care physicians, most personal health needs are appropriately and efficiently handled by a patient's primary care physician.

As the first point of contact, primary care physicians initially address all problems and health questions that patients may have. While it is unfortunately not common knowledge in the general public, primary care physicians have no restriction as to the problems or organ systems that they address, and they are comfortable diagnosing and treating acute illnesses, chronic disease processes, and the most common injuries.

Primary care physicians are experts in all common physical, mental, emotional, and social concerns. They have the appropriate training to manage a large majority of problems in their offices and only involve specialists for further evaluation or treatment when requested by the patient or when it is deemed necessary by the physician and in the best interest of the patient.

## 2. Provide Continuity and Accountability

Primary care physicians uniquely provide continuity of medical care and accountability to their patients for their current and long-term health. Specifically, this benefit of primary care is the continuity that comes from an ongoing relationship and rapport with a physician who knows their patients' entire health and personal history. Over multiple years treating the patient, the physician develops a context for optimal care and possesses an accumulated personal health record to better evaluate each new concern and manage any chronic conditions.

As, inevitably, patients require some specialty care by other physicians and healthcare providers, their primary physician makes referrals, is aware of the assessments and treatments by the specialists, coordinates care of multiple providers as needed, and (maybe most importantly) serves as a translator for complicated and technical information and medical terminology that specialists may not have time to communicate adequately to the patient.

In addition, the primary care physician assumes a proactive role of responsibility and accountability for ongoing care and decision-making about their patients' health, self-care, preventive care, and ongoing medical management. In optimal circumstances decision-making and accountability are shared with the patient in a very real sense. This kind of ongoing relationship with a primary care physician over the years is invaluable and cannot be approximated by isolated encounters with telemedicine or urgent care doctors.

## *3. Address Proactive Preventive Care*

Primary care physicians know that longevity and quality of life are directly linked to proactive preventive care. Patients who are engaged in a long-term relationship with a primary care physician are more likely to be advised about and pursue healthy lifestyle choices, risk factor reduction measures, and timely screening for hidden medical risks and impending medical conditions. In most cases, these disease prevention and early detection measures have a greater impact on overall health than do interventions for acute illnesses.

HEALTH RISK MODIFICATION: Periodic discussions about health goals with this trusted medical adviser allow patients to understand health risks better and encourage them to make lifestyle choices that are proven to improve quality of life and delay or prevent a myriad of medical disorders. It is common knowledge that tobacco use (smoking, chewing, and now nicotine-containing vaping), excessive alcohol consumption, illicit drug use, poor diet, lack of exercise, and overweight/obesity are the leading modifiable risk factors for disease and premature death.

Doctors know that pills are easy and lifestyle changes are hard. The value that primary care physicians provide are centered around personalized explanations about the reasons that healthy lifestyle prolongs life, the importance and impact of patients' choices, advice on practical tips to making change happen, and repeated encouragement over time.

TIMELY PREVENTIVE SCREENINGS: Another major area of preventive care is screening for hidden disease and risk. The primary care physician advises and reminds patients concerning preventive screening guidelines that, when followed, result in early detection of disease and improved health outcomes.

Research has shown that regular primary care visits are associated with an increase in recommended preventive interventions including an increase of 127% for vaccinations, 122% for colonoscopy, and 75% for mammography. Many categories of health screenings are recommended based on the patient's age and existing risks. Screenings of patients who are completely without symptoms frequently uncover issues related to virtually every organ system and significant medical conditions. People who do not undergo these screenings often have advanced issues including cardiovascular diseases, cancers, metabolic conditions, and countless other potentially life-threatening problems by the time symptoms are present and diagnosed.

## 4. Help Patients Navigate the Healthcare System

The American healthcare system is complex and confusing. Individuals who have a reliable relationship with and timely access to a primary care physician are more likely to utilize healthcare services appropriately, efficiently, and cost-effectively. Utilizing their primary care physician as a health services concierge, they are less likely to require secondary care from specialists including emergency room visits, urgent care, telemedicine services (with an unknown doctor/nurse), or care delivered by various specialist physicians.

Patients who first consulted their primary care physician are also felt to have utilized emergency department care less often for COVID-19 concerns. The physician educates their patients about recommended facilities for ancillary services (imaging, physical therapy, sleep labs, for example) and advises them about cost-effective approaches to purchasing prescription medications, among other health-related direction.

There is an alarming variation in prices for medical services among various facilities. Imaging studies such as x-rays, CT scans, and MRIs may often be obtained for cash prices that are significantly less than many patients' copayments under their insurance plans. And simply by making effective prescription medication choices and coaching their patients on how to receive discounted cash pricing on their medications, primary care physicians may save their patients more than the total cost the physician charges for delivering their care.

## *5. Provide Better Health with Lower Cost*

Reliable access to primary care has proven to result in improved health outcomes and overall healthcare cost savings. Better access to primary care and a greater number of primary care physicians in a geographic area are associated with improved health status and lower mortality rates.

Multiple studies performed across the United States have shown a consistent relationship between the ratio of primary care physicians to the population as the only consistent predictor of age-specific mortality rates, and mortality associated with cancer, heart disease, neonatal mortality, and life expectancy.

While delivering improved health outcomes, primary care is widely recognized to simultaneously reduce overall healthcare costs by means of all the benefits listed in this chapter. Healthcare costs go down when medical conditions are detected early and managed efficiently by primary care physicians. Costs also go down when unnecessary overutilization of expensive specialty and emergency care is contained or eliminated and when care is delivered by the least expensive medical providers and institutions. Primary care is inherently less expensive than the care delivered by specialty physicians and institutions that provide secondary and specialty care.

## From My Practice

When some people reach a certain age and have struggled with more medical issues than they would like, they feel like they are continually going to doctors and spending their money on medical services and products. It can be said that your degree of health is inversely proportional to the number of doctors that you know. Having too many doctors means that you have too many medical problems. In my medical practice, I have seen this phenomenon many times. Fortunately, as a primary care physician managing a broad range of medical conditions, I can often help simplify the medical lives of my patients.

Matt had too many doctors. Being sixty-one and overweight, he had developed several medical problems that are so common that they are almost predictable. These issues had led him to seek care with several specialist physicians. He was seeing a cardiologist who managed his high blood pressure and cholesterol, a pulmonologist sleep specialist who prescribed a CPAP machine for his sleep apnea, and a urologist to get medication for his urinary symptoms due to an enlarged prostate. In addition to these doctors, he saw an allergist once or twice per year when over-the-counter medications weren't keeping his seasonal allergy symptoms in check, and he had landed at one of those "low T" clinics where he was receiving weekly testosterone shots.

Even with all of these doctors in his life, any time he would get sick or experience a minor injury, he would run up to the nearby urgent care clinic where he could be seen by a random doctor or nurse practitioner. As if all of those doctor visits weren't enough, the prescriptions from his specialist physicians were often brand-name drugs that were very expensive, even with his insurance. Matt certainly felt like his healthcare ruled his life.

He found out about my medical practice from a friend. Matt's friend told him that (much to his surprise) there are doctors who are available when you need them and partner with you in managing the majority of medical needs that you may have. From my initial meeting with Matt it was obvious that every one of his medical issues was common and simple for a primary care physician to manage. We primary care doctors consider ourselves specialists in common conditions.

Matt and I discussed his previously diagnosed conditions and agreed that I would take over the care and prescriptions for his high blood pressure, high cholesterol, sleep apnea, obesity, prostatic hyperplasia (enlarged prostate), seasonal allergies, low testosterone as well as promising to be available whenever he needed me to address any illnesses or injuries that might come up. He fired all of his specialists! Why use five doctors when one will do?

In addition to freeing up a lot of time and copayments that he used to spend at all of those doctors, it was obvious that there were better and more cost-effective ways to manage Matt's medications. One of the problems with multiple doctors prescribing multiple medications is that no single physician is coordinating care and ensuring that each of those medications is working best with the others (not to mention being aware of the total bill that the patient is paying for medicines that he has been asked to take by his other doctors!).

I switched him to highly effective generic medications for the conditions that needed to be treated, taught him how he could find discounts online for his prescription medicines to be used at his local pharmacy that would allow him to pay cash (without insurance) and pay far less than the amount that he was responsible for if he were to run those purchases through his pharmacy benefits insurance. This simple change saved him far more than the total amount he pays for my services every year.

## A Trusted Adviser

Primary care is the logical foundation of healthcare. It is the best and most efficient first stop for immediate needs (illness and injury) as well as for the diagnosis and long-term management of most diseases and other medical conditions. Beyond those interventions, primary care is also the most likely setting for patient education and accountability related to health risk reduction and preventive care—the elements of healthcare that have the greatest impact on health and longevity throughout people's lives.

A relationship with a personal primary care physician over time is a virtual necessity for anyone who wants to receive the most valuable elements of our modern healthcare system in an efficient and caring manner.

You need a doctor. Primary care physicians can provide the most personal, effective, and economical of all medical care. But there's a problem. The traditional systems for the delivery of primary care in the United States have become inefficient and are challenging to navigate, both for patients and their doctors. In Part II of this book, I'll look at why gaining reliable access to your primary care physician has become so difficult.

# PART II

# WHY IS GETTING THE MEDICAL CARE I NEED SO FRUSTRATING?

# 4

# The Current State of Primary Care in America

The current state of primary care in America is . . . frustration. For numerous reasons, the delivery of primary care services and access to primary care physicians have become increasingly difficult and frustrating. Who hasn't asked themselves all of these questions?

- Why can't I just get my doctor on the phone for two minutes?
- Wouldn't it be so much easier if I could simply text my doctor a question?
- Why can't I schedule an appointment to see my doctor today?
- What am I supposed to do at night or on the weekend when my doctor's office is closed and I have a medical issue?

- Why do I have to schedule a different appointment for every problem I need to address?
- Why can't I see the same doctor every time I come in?
- Why do I have to see a nurse practitioner or physician assistant instead of my doctor?
- Why is the doctor so rushed?
- Why doesn't the doctor listen?
- Why is my doctor always running way behind schedule?
- Why do I have to fill out all this paperwork every time I go to the doctor's office?

The fact is, the delivery system for primary care in America is overly taxed to the point that access to primary care physicians and the quality of care are suffering. There are several reasons for this current state and more than a few measurable negative consequences of it. Too many people are not connected with a personal physician over time and are not receiving many of the benefits of primary care that I have been discussing so far.

It is clear that better delivery of primary care would improve population health and decrease costs. Unfortunately, the exact opposite is occurring and seems likely to worsen. Currently, 82 million people in the US (a full 25% of the population) do not have anyone that they recognize as their primary care physician. Sadly, 20% of adults have not seen any doctor within the past year, and only 8% have received all recommended high-priority preventive services.

More recently, nearly 40% of Americans have avoided doctor visits for important medical symptoms and preventive services during the COVID-19 pandemic due to concerns about not feeling safe going to the office. This current inadequate state of primary care is driven by several factors:

- An increasing shortage of primary care physicians
- With fewer doctors, those in practice are overextended
- Ongoing effects of the COVID-19 pandemic
- Clearly negative effects of health insurance participation in the relationship between primary care physicians and their patients

These factors result in poor quality of care, low patient satisfaction with access to primary care, and an ever-increasing cost of care. I discuss each of these factors in detail over the next three chapters.

## Shortage of Primary Care Physicians

America is experiencing a shortage of primary care physicians. You may have experienced this in delays in access, long wait times, rushed appointments, physician sentiment concerning their practices, and complaints from the general public that they find it difficult to find a doctor.

Research conducted in September 2019 by Public Opinion Strategies indicated that 35% of respondents had trouble finding a doctor over the preceding three years and, according to a 2017 study by Merritt Hawkins, the national average cumulative wait time to schedule a new patient-physician appointment is twenty-four days—the longest it has been since the survey began in 2004.

The rapid expansion of physician extenders or midlevel providers across the country is further evidence of a demand for medical services that substantially exceeds the capacity of our currently licensed physician workforce. Nonphysician providers are typically trained and licensed as physician assistants and nurse practitioners who provide care under the supervision of physicians.

There are currently over 325,000 nurse practitioners (NPs) and more than 115,000 Certified Physician Assistants (PAs) practicing in the United States. Of these, about 27% of PAs and 75% of NPs are providing primary care services. That equates to about 275,000 midlevel providers, which is nearly as many as the 299,000 practicing primary care physicians.

Prior to the rise of COVID-19, the magnitude of the primary care physician shortage had been estimated at 55,000 physicians nationwide by 2033. In addition to the recent effect that the pandemic has had on disruption of primary care, the main drivers of this shortage are an aging population, accelerated physician retirement, and a low percentage of new physicians choosing to specialize in primary care.

## *Demographics*

The US population aged sixty-five and older is projected to grow by 45.1% by the year 2033. As our elderly population continues to grow, the demand for general and specialty physician care is also expected to increase dramatically. It is self-apparent that the older we get, the more likely we are to require healthcare services. Older adults use far more healthcare services than younger adults and children.

The diagnosis of serious or chronic health problems increases with age and is directly associated with higher per capita healthcare costs. Specifically, people over the age of fifty-five make up 29% of the population but account for 56% of all health spending. The declining health and increasing healthcare costs that occur with age increase the workload for physicians practicing primary care and also for specialist physicians. To compound matters, at the same time that patients are aging and requiring more care, their physicians are aging and may be less able to deliver the same volume of care.

## *Physician Retirement*

The baby boomers are retiring. Baby boomer physicians are now retiring at an accelerated rate. Greater than 40% of currently active physicians will be at traditional retirement age of sixty-five or older within the next decade, including myself, at the same time that baby boomer patients are requiring more care. Additionally, physician surveys indicate that 31.6% of practicing primary care physicians are currently experiencing anxiety, withdrawal, and burnout, which is likely to result in significantly earlier retirement than has occurred historically.

There seems to also be an ongoing effect of COVID-19 on physician practice patterns and their attitudes about retirement. The added stresses and financial concerns that have occurred with the COVID-19 pandemic have led some primary care physicians to early retirement—yet another unexpected consequence of the pandemic. A survey of primary care physicians conducted in September 2020 indicated that 19% of respondents experienced physicians in their practice retiring or planning to retire due directly to the consequences of the COVID-19 pandemic.

## *Fewer Physicians Choosing Primary Care*

At the same time that older physicians are retiring (some earlier than expected), new physicians are not choosing primary care. Physicians graduating from medical school have a lot of options when it comes to choosing an area of medicine to pursue as their career. Their interests, lifestyles, work-life balance, and income are greatly impacted by this choice.

The number and percentage of medical school graduates who are pursuing careers in primary care have dropped dramatically over the past thirty years. From 1997 to 2005, the number of US medical graduates entering family medicine residencies dropped by 50%, and according to the 2019 Residency Match Report, only 41% of available internal medicine residency positions were filled by MD students graduating from US medical schools. Similar trends were seen in family medicine and pediatrics. The percentage of active physicians practicing primary care in the US has decreased from 50% in 1961 to less than 32% in 2019.

The financial ramifications of choosing a career in primary care are a significant factor in the declining interest in primary care careers. There is a substantial compensation gap between primary care and specialty physicians. The highest earning specialist physicians average twice the annual salary of primary care physicians. This, in conjunction with the significantly increasing cost of medical education, has made primary care relatively unattractive from a financial standpoint.

Physicians simply do not wish to accept lower salaries and income when faced with a quarter of a million dollars in medical school debt.

## Primary Care under Pressure

From the primary care physicians' standpoint, they are under increasing pressure from all sides and for many reasons. Demands on doctors come from patients, third parties (most often payers that are health insurance companies), employers, and, when self-employed, from the rising administrative costs of operating a medical practice.

As previously discussed, increasing patient demand in the face of waning primary care physician supply causes doctors to be overextended. Their appointment schedules are overbooked or double-booked and extend for long hours caring for patients in their offices. Of course, a schedule that is beyond reasonable capacity does not leave any time to care for patients who have important questions and medical needs but are not physically in the office. That, along with historically lower reimbursement by insurance companies for remote over-the-phone care, is the reason you can rarely talk with your doctor via telephone for even the simplest matter.

This consistently high-volume workload creates a constant source of pressure that physicians must manage while attempting to stay on schedule and seeking to avoid frustrating their patients when they don't. Primary care doctors are forced to rush through patient visits. They have no choice but to abbreviate the time that they take listening to patients and asking important questions, which predictably frustrates both the doctor and the patient and drives physician job stress.

The vast majority of primary care physicians, whether in privately owned practices or as employees of large physician groups or hospitals, are paid based on reimbursement by their patients' medical insurance. There is a pressure to bill for more services and collect more in reimbursement in order to improve the profitability of the private practice or the hospital/hospital system that may employ them. Often, direct pressure is exerted on physicians to be more productive. Of course, productivity relates to the volume of patients seen and services rendered but only if insurance companies consider them covered services and reimburse the medical practice.

In order to provide payment, these third parties require physicians to document all patient encounters and services rendered via large amounts of descriptive documentation and standardized coding of procedures/services rendered and diagnoses established. Physicians carry the pressure of this documentation as it is the only way they are paid for their work. If their documentation does not meet the expectations of the insurance company, payment will be denied or delayed.

At the same time, the complexity and volume of documentation and coding required to satisfy third-party payers has increased dramatically since the passage of the Affordable Care Act in 2010. This healthcare law affected both Medicare and private health insurance carriers and has resulted in additional pressure on physicians in primary care practice.

Another area of pressure being experienced by primary care physicians is the increasing cost to run a medical practice. The administrative overhead of medical practices is going up. Costs for medical practices are increasing due to the increasing costs to comply with the requirements for private health insurance reimbursement, Medicare, and the Affordable Care Act even as reimbursement rates have remained flat. The costs of support staff, technology (required by law and payers), legal and regulatory expenses, and office space are also on the rise.

For physicians who own their own practices and are participating providers with major health insurance carriers, the only means to offset increasing practice costs is by increasing the volume of patients seen by each doctor, along with the number of tests and treatments performed. This dynamic further feeds the high-volume-based model that puts pressure on physicians and frustrates patients. The pressure of increasing practice overhead along with flat reimbursement rates for their services have resulted in inconsistent income for physicians in private practice and have driven many primary care physicians to become employees of hospital systems or large physician practices.

As of 2018, there are now more employed physicians than physician practice owners, and family physicians are the specialty with the greatest percentage practicing as employed physicians (57.4%).

Whether in private practice or as employees of hospitals, primary care physicians see an average of twenty patients per day (with 14% seeing thirty to sixty patients per day) in order to earn about half the income of many specialists. If you're one of the thirty patients leafing through old magazines in the waiting room, you know about the wait time for a precious few minutes with a physician.

Not surprisingly, a survey by The Physicians Foundation found that 81% of doctors describe themselves as either overextended or at full capacity, and 39% said they planned to cut back on the number of patients they see, accelerate their retirement plans, work part-time, or close their practices to new patients.

In July 2020 a national survey of physicians indicated that the additional demands placed on physicians by the COVID-19 pandemic had resulted in a reduction of income (72% of respondents), reduced office staff (43%), practice closure (8%), and a belief by 59% of physicians that the

COVID-19 pandemic will lead to a reduction in the number of independent physician practices in their communities.

## Patient Experience

You might have heard the term *patient experience* related to healthcare services and assumed it simply means *customer satisfaction*. While the terms are closely linked and may overlap, they are different. Patient experience, as defined by the Agency for Healthcare Research and Quality (AHRQ) is this:

> [E]ncompasses the range of interactions that patients have with the health care system, including their care from health plans, and from doctors, nurses, and staff in hospitals, physician practices, and other health care facilities. As an integral component of health care quality, patient experience includes several aspects of health care delivery that patients value highly when they seek and receive care, such as getting timely appointments, easy access to information, and good communication with health care providers.

Patient satisfaction is more subjective. Patient satisfaction refers to whether a patient's expectations about a doctor's visit or medical service encounter were met. Patient experience measures are more objective indicators of quality of care. For you to receive excellent care and to be happy about it, you will need to receive both at a high level.

The current state of patient experience and patient satisfaction in America related to primary care leave much to be desired. While you don't think of it in terms of patient experience, any frustrations you have with patient satisfaction and service are likely diminishing your quality of care and patient experience as well. Surveys of patient satisfaction show that 95% of people who have a primary care physician like them and trust their advice. However, the majority of patients surveyed are dissatisfied with their level of customer service and access to their physician.

A 2013 study by Consumer Reports National Research Center indicated the following problems were most frequent and most bothersome to patients:

- Excessive delay in obtaining an appointment when ill
- Limited time with their doctor who appears rushed during office visit
- Long wait for the doctor after arriving at their office
- Difficulty reaching their doctor by phone or email

The issue of high demand on the time of primary care physicians who are in shorter supply has resulted in an average patient panel (the number of patients that each doctor is responsible to care for) estimated in the range of 2,300 patients per physician, an average wait time in the office of more than twenty minutes, a majority of visits less than sixteen minutes with the doctor and a twenty-four-day delay for a new patient to receive an office visit.

What do you want from a doctor? If you're like most people, you really want answers from your doctor, and you want them now. You want to know the answers to the questions *What's wrong with me?* and *What should I do about it?* You want to be able to reach your doctor over the phone or to see them in their office on the same day whenever you have the need. You don't want to have to wait. You do want enough time with your doctor to fully explain what's going on and what you think is important. The doctor needs to be patient and listen. They also have to be willing to sit and explain your problem, your test results, your diagnosis, and their treatment recommendations.

If you don't get all of that consistently over time, you will be frustrated. You will not have a good patient experience, will not receive good customer service, and will not have high patient satisfaction with your care. Unfortunately, disappointment in many of these areas is all too common.

## From My Practice

Let me tell you a story about a physician friend of mine. I believe her story and frustrations with the progression of her career as a primary care physician will give you some insight into the current state of primary care in America and why you may be frustrated trying to get what you need from your doctor.

Amanda joined a small privately owned family practice with just two other doctors in 1992, shortly after finishing her residency. It was a busy practice, but she always prioritized spending time with her patients and was able to see patients when they needed her. They appreciated it, referred their friends and family, and the practice grew.

Amanda got busy. The practice hired more staff, then more physicians, then more middle managers. The overhead of the practice was going up faster than the reimbursement by insurance carriers for the doctors' services. Then, in 2010, the Affordable Care Act became law. Compliance with the act, along with additional requirements from insurance companies in order to be paid, and apprehension about the potential sustainability of the practice and their income led the physician-owners to sell their practice to a large and expanding hospital system in their region of the country.

The sale of Amanda's medical practice certainly didn't make her rich, but she was okay with it. Amanda was hopeful that without the pressures of managing and owning the practice, she could focus on doing what she went into medicine for in the first place. As an employee of the hospital, maybe she could spend more time with her patients and deliver compassionate and higher quality care.

As it turned out, the hospital administration had other ideas. She was required to attend weekly meetings reviewing the performance of the practice and working on plans to improve its capacity, productivity, and contribution to the hospital's bottom line. She also had regular reviews of her personal billing practices and productivity. Amanda was regularly pressured by the hospital administrators to change her appointment schedule, accommodate more patients, see them faster, bill more services, and make more referrals for tests, specialist consultations, and admissions to the hospital and its affiliates.

The move she felt she had to make to become an employed physician had not simplified her life. Far from it. This change also caused many of her longtime patients to become more frustrated with their lack of access to Amanda since she was scheduled beyond a reasonable capacity and was always in a hurry. This very common progression for primary care physicians to become hospital employees only compounded the issues currently being faced by so many doctors and their patients.

## The Frustrating Treadmill of Primary Care

Efficient delivery of primary care by an adequate number of physicians practicing under a model that allows them the time to know their patients, be available when needed, and interact with them when not in a rush would result in healthier and happier patients with a high level of satisfaction with care and a low level of frustration with the healthcare system.

Unfortunately, the typical insurance-based primary care delivery system in the US is headed in the opposite direction. The current overtaxed primary care system and corresponding lack of access to primary care physicians deters people from seeking care in a timely manner for medical symptoms and from receiving important preventive screenings. This results in an excess number of people who live with undiagnosed and untreated medical conditions that decrease their quality and duration of life and eventually require more costly emergency and specialty care.

Together, health outcomes, patient satisfaction with care, and healthcare costs are all negatively affected by the current state of primary care. COVID-19 threw an additional wrench in the works. America and the world are on the heels of a pandemic that has further degraded our primary care delivery system. In the next chapter I consider short-term, medium-term, and long-term effects of COVID-19 on primary care.

# 5

# Consequences of COVID-19 on Primary Care

The COVID-19 pandemic affected us all. It affected the delivery of primary care dramatically.

On the backdrop of an overly taxed primary care delivery system, with declining supply of providers, increasing pressure on physicians, and low patient satisfaction with access, the COVID-19 pandemic further impacted the delivery of primary care in several ways. At the beginning of the pandemic in the United States as travel, business, and personal contact were suddenly restricted, primary care practices drastically restricted in-person appointment slots and struggled to adapt to a version of telemedicine. Prior to the pandemic, only 18% of primary care physicians had offered any telemedicine services.

Another significant impact on primary care practices in the early days of the pandemic was financial. Physician practices are fee-for-service businesses that are almost exclusively compensated by insurance companies for in-person medical services. Therefore, the pandemic caused doctors' incomes to plummet as patient visits to primary care offices were minimized. As the pandemic progressed, the challenges to primary care practices and their patients seeking care evolved.

The medium-term and long-term impact of COVID-19 on primary care is still being realized and analyzed more than a year and a half into the pandemic. By the summer of 2020, physicians were starting to better understand the behavior of the virus—how it made us sick, best approaches for treating severe infections, and most likely ways to mitigate or reduce the spread of the virus. This included safety policies within doctors' offices as well as personal safety concepts of mask wearing, handwashing, and social distancing.

Another consequence realized during this time was patients' substantial avoidance of medical care. Fear of contracting COVID at medical facilities kept people from seeking very important medical care, including care for acute medical conditions as well as routine and preventive services.

Finally, the long-term or permanent effects of the pandemic are real but remain to be fully quantified. There are currently more questions than answers about the long-term effects on people's health due to the avoidance of care for over a year or more and also the ways that our healthcare system will have been changed for the better or worse during this global health crisis.

## Immediate Short-Term Impact

In the early days of the COVID-19 pandemic, primary care came to a screeching, almost complete stop.

On January 9, 2020, the World Health Organization announced fifty-nine cases of a mysterious coronavirus-related pneumonia in Wuhan, China, and the first case of the 2019 novel coronavirus was confirmed in the United States by the CDC on January 15, 2020. By January 31 the WHO had declared a global public health emergency, followed three days later by the US declaration of a national health emergency.

COVID-19 was designated a pandemic by WHO on March 11, and on March 16 President Donald Trump, in conjunction with the CDC, issued coronavirus guidelines, which encouraged Americans to limit their normal behaviors and interactions for "15 days to slow the spread." These guidelines initiated a cascade of guidance from federal, state, and local health officials and various legal mandates at all levels of government, which resulted in lockdowns of many aspects of American life. Access to primary care doctors and healthcare in general through the typical means were no exception.

As the threat of COVID-19 became obvious, primary care practices immediately took action to protect their patients and staff against the transmission of the virus. Many practices closed their doors or screened all patients by phone to determine how to triage their care. Since community physicians did not have access to testing for the SARS-CoV-2 virus at that time or any known treatments, severely ill patients were told to go to hospital emergency departments for care.

If they were not severely ill, they were instructed to stay home and to isolate away from other people for a couple of weeks and until symptoms had resolved. Primary care physicians understandably avoided in-office visits whenever possible. Little was known about the virus in the spring of 2020, and most primary care practices were not equipped with protective equipment (personal protective equipment or PPE was not a commonly used term in primary practice at the time, let alone in the general public) presumed to be necessary to keep their patients and staff from contracting COVID-19 infection.

Offices postponed all preventive visits, most visits for management of chronic diseases, and, whenever possible, visits for illnesses and injuries in order to avoid the risk of contributing to additional spread. Also, as expected, patients were not only afraid of contracting COVID in their everyday lives, but they aggressively avoided care in physicians' offices and also at hospital emergency rooms, fearing they would catch the virus by coming into contact with other sick patients who were seeking medical care.

These lockdowns of primary care practices and social distancing (another term not in use prior to the pandemic) led to a new interest in expanding the use of remote care and telemedicine.

Prior to COVID-19, the vast majority of Medicare recipients were prohibited from utilizing telemedicine services, and the majority of private insurers either did not cover remote care or reimbursed these services at substantially lower rates than in-person office visits and services. Since the vast majority of primary care and other physicians are contractually participating providers with Medicare and private insurance carriers and these third-party payers were not covering telemedicine services, doctors' offices were not offering any meaningful virtual services to their patients.

On March 26, 2020, the Senate passed the CARES Act, which included a provision that allowed the Centers for Medicare & Medicaid Services (CMS) to waive the rule limiting the use of telehealth services, but only in cases where a prior established doctor-patient relationship existed. Again, private insurers followed suit and also began to expand coverage for telemedicine services and virtual visits. In the early stages of the pandemic, most primary care practices were not equipped to efficiently schedule and deliver services remotely via video chat and had to adapt to even provide a significant amount of their services via phone.

The pandemic also produced immediate and dire financial consequences on primary care practices. As the vast majority of primary care physicians practice in an insurance-participating, fee-for-service, volume-based business model, the sudden drop in patient visits and corresponding diagnostic tests and treatments hit them as hard as restaurants that had no patrons. As discussed in the previous chapter, privately owned primary care practices were already under substantial economic pressure prior to COVID, and within a few short months of the start of the pandemic, their financial situations worsened.

A nationwide survey conducted by The Physicians Foundation in August 2020 found these alarming statistics:

- 8% of physicians had closed their practices as a result of COVID-19.
- Of physicians who closed their practices, 76% were private practice owners or partners.
- 43% of physicians had reduced their staff due to COVID-19.
- 72% of physicians had experienced a reduction of income due to COVID-19.
- 41% of physicians saw a decrease in volume of services of greater than 25%.
- 12% had switched to a primarily telemedicine practice due to COVID-19.

- 59% of physicians believed COVID-19 would lead to a decrease in independent physician practices in their communities.

Another survey conducted around the same time found that 7% of primary care practices were not confident that they could remain in business past the end of 2020 without financial assistance. While many medical practices availed themselves of forgivable loans through the federal Paycheck Protection Program (PPP), the financial shortfall of their practices remained devastating. A study by Harvard Medical School and the American Board of Family Medicine estimated the potential impact of COVID-19 on primary care practices in the US for the calendar year 2020 at $15.1 billion and found that this number could more than double if telemedicine payment policies enacted during COVID-19 were not sustained.

## Medium-Term Impact

The summer and fall of 2020 brought a better understanding of the behavior of the SARS-CoV-2 virus and stark realization of the ongoing effects that the pandemic would have on our health, livelihoods, and traffic patterns, and on the delivery of healthcare in our country. Medical observations and research began to give us an understanding of how the virus was most likely to spread, how contagious it was and how deadly.

During March 2020, many hospital systems were offering COVID-19 testing and by mid-April 2020, the Food and Drug Administration (FDA) had approved 117 diagnostic tests including PCR, serological antibody tests, isothermal RNA tests, and, later, antigen tests. Many of these quickly received Emergency Use Authorization and became available for use on patients at hospitals, at diagnostic labs, and in pop-up testing facilities.

The ability for primary care practices to test for COVID infection made mitigation efforts and recommendations concerning treatment, quarantines, and isolation much more effective. Most primary care practices eventually developed the ability to perform certain COVID tests on-site or to obtain specimens that were sent to diagnostic labs in order to direct the care of their patients.

Unfortunately, even as the medical community had better information about COVID-19 and office policies in place to protect their patients, fear about the virus continued to keep many people from seeking medical care of all kinds. By the end of June, the CDC estimated that 41% of US adults had avoided medical care because of concerns about COVID-19. This included 12% who avoided urgent or emergency care, and 32% who avoided routine care.

Further, delaying or avoiding emergency care was even more common in people with disabilities and those with two or more underlying health conditions. In another June 2020 health tracking poll, 27% of those who skipped or postponed medical care reported that they subsequently experienced a worsening of their medical condition(s). The consequences of this avoidance of care—specifically the disruptions to the management of chronic diseases and other routine nonemergent care—may be even more significant than we currently suspect.

In addition to the likely effect on the physical health of people who postpone or skip important medical care altogether, the pandemic has had a significant and documented effect on the developmental and emotional health of Americans.

Widespread negative effects on people's employment and income, business viability, education and career disruption as well as their normal socialization and traffic patterns have resulted in increases in feelings of fear, clinical anxiety, and depression, which have led to increased suicide and crime rates, among other negative consequences.

Declines in mental health in conjunction with the pandemic have affected many Americans but have been most pronounced in certain groups: 56% of young adults (ages eighteen to twenty-four) report anxiety or depression that they attributed to the pandemic during 2020. Adults in households that experienced job loss in connection with COVID-19 were significantly more likely than those without job loss or loss of income to report mental illness (53% vs. 32%).

Throughout the pandemic, 47% of women described symptoms of anxiety or depression compared with 38% of men as of December 2020. Adolescents were hard hit, not only in terms of anxiety and depression but in rates of substance use, suicidal ideations, and suicide as well. According to the CDC, young children (birth to five years) also experienced a broad indirect negative impact on their social, emotional, and mental well-being as a result of the changes in routine, interruption of care and education, missed significant life events, a loss of security and safety as well as a break in the continuity of their healthcare.

In the medium-term of six to twelve months into the pandemic, primary care practices attempted to return to a version of normal. They became more prepared and comfortable seeing a greater number of patients in their offices and opened their appointment schedules accordingly. At the same time, more patients realized that it was not a good idea to continue to avoid going to the doctor for medical symptoms and management of their chronic conditions or to further postpone preventive care and check-ups—thus creating a backlog of demand for primary care services and a return to the prepandemic strain on doctors and their offices. Of course, patients again experienced a return to the status quo of challenges in securing timely access to their doctors.

## Permanent (Long-Term) Effects

A significant percentage of the US population is now either vaccinated or possessing natural immunity due to past COVID-19 infection, and in spite of ongoing spread of the virus and its variants (as well as hospitalizations and deaths primarily in the unvaccinated), the worst of the pandemic seems to be behind us.

And while most virologists and epidemiologists believe that the SARS-CoV-2 and its variants will continue to be with us to some degree into the foreseeable future, it is likely that, going forward, we will consider it much more like the seasonal flu than a societal risk that necessitates drastic modification of our daily lives. Nevertheless, the aftermath of this pandemic may be with us in many ways for years to come.

The temporary changes in lifestyle and the utilization of important healthcare services during at least sixteen months of the pandemic had a measurable effect on the physical and emotional health of many Americans. What remains to be calculated is the degree that these negative consequences will be with us years down the road. We will continue to ask these questions and observe the outcomes:

- Will a year of weight gain and disruption of some healthy habits or avoidance of disease management for diabetes, high blood pressure, high cholesterol, heart conditions, and others shorten our lives?

- How many people developed life-threatening medical conditions during the pandemic that were not diagnosed in a timely manner, leading to worse outcomes due to avoidance of preventive screenings? How many mammograms and colonoscopies were postponed?
- Will students who endured the disruption of two school years recover what they missed academically and socially?
- How about the many adolescents that became further dependent on their smartphones and escalated already alarming rates of anxiety, depression, chemical dependency, and suicide?

While we may believe our health as a society has returned to normal when we no longer hear about COVID-19 deaths, we need to be on the lookout for the lingering effects of this rare and unique health crisis.

There is another question that has not yet been answered: Will there be long-term effects on the delivery of primary care services due to the COVID-19 pandemic?

It seems that there will. Concerns about physician burnout lead many to believe that the shortage of primary care physicians previously discussed will worsen due to decisions by more primary care physicians to retire early at least in part due to their experiences throughout the pandemic.

A further shortage of primary care physicians in America will be difficult to overcome with future medical school graduates, and a higher percentage of primary care services are likely to be delivered by midlevel nurse practitioners and physician assistants rather than by licensed physicians. Midlevel providers serve a crucial role as practice extenders under the supervision of physicians, but most people I speak with recognize the value of the additional training and experience that physicians could provide if a shortage did not exist.

Another highly impactful influence on the delivery of primary care that is likely to be affected by COVID for years to come is the reimbursement environment and health insurance involvement in primary care. The executive order waiver included in the CARES Act that has allowed for Medicare reimbursement of telemedicine services is not currently permanent. Unless permanent legislation is enacted securing the provision of remote care, the trend toward the use of efficient virtual care for many conditions may be in jeopardy.

Finally, it remains to be seen whether an increased number of primary care physicians will actually retire as a result of COVID or if patients' experiences during the pandemic will cause them to demand better access to primary care within newer delivery models that guarantee them access to their doctors whenever they need them.

## From My Practice

By the time the World Health Organization and President Trump declared global and national health emergencies at the end of January 2020, it was obvious that the COVID-19 pandemic would substantially affect all Americans and all businesses, including healthcare businesses. Primary care practices would need to change the way they delivered care to their patients. When nationwide mitigation recommendations were put forward by the CDC and the President in mid-March 2020, it was obvious that the shutdown would be honored to a significant degree by doctors' offices.

In my small primary care practice in the Kansas City area, we immediately modified the way we delivered care. We quickly developed and enacted COVID-19 safety policies and procedures and announced them to our patients. We reminded them that the safety and well-being of our patients and staff would remain our top priority. They could rest assured that in the midst of uncertainty surrounding the spread of the coronavirus, they would continue to have access to their personal physician. Our practice was already providing our patients with unrestricted, 24/7 direct access to their doctor by phone, text, email, and secure patient portal, which made this transition much easier for our patients than most.

Throughout the pandemic, we promised our patients that our physicians would closely monitor the announcements and guidance of federal, state, and local health authorities for handling risk, potential exposure, and treatment of the coronavirus and would maintain policies that were consistent with their guidance and the mandates of government.

Our practice policies evolved along with the progression of the pandemic. For about the first eight weeks following the March 16 announcement of "15 days to slow the spread," we paused all but the most urgent in-office appointments but provided an increased and high volume of virtual care via phone, video chat, text, email, and secure portal messaging. We canceled all preventive visits and performed phone screening for every patient requesting an appointment. If any recognizable risk for COVID-19 was identified, patients were scheduled for virtual visits with their doctor who addressed their medical concern and either provided treatment over the phone, asked them to come to our office, or advised them of another course of action (such as "go to the ER").

Our in-office patient visits dropped to near zero, but we were able to retain all staff, paying them full-time pay for working half-time. In addition, aggressive in-office infection control measures were put in place. Over time, we began to see more patients in our office, continued to screen for symptoms of illness prior to appointments, kept patients isolated and out of the waiting room, and utilized full personal protective equipment as advised by the CDC.

As the pandemic progressed, we continued to follow the guidance for healthcare facilities. We initially referred patients to hospital testing facilities, then obtained specimens curbside in our parking lot to send to an outside diagnostic lab, and ultimately were able to also offer rapid antigen testing on-site for certain patients who would benefit from it.

In January and February of 2021, every staff member in our office was vaccinated and by April vaccines were widely available to the general public. Our practice has been busy as we caught up on preventive screenings and check-ups that were postponed throughout the pandemic. We have been encouraging more than a few people to reverse some of the unhealthy habits they developed while working from home and to take off their COVID twenty (pounds).

Our practice grew during the pandemic. Because of our unique business model and the high level of direct access we provide as each patient's personal physician, our patients regularly told us that they were so glad they were patients of our practice during this unprecedented health crisis and that simply being able to get answers now from a doctor they knew and trusted was invaluable.

## COVID Aftershocks

COVID-19 affected us all. For the majority of Americans who did not contract severe coronavirus disease, require hospitalization, experience death among their friends or family, and haven't been one of those with persistent long-hauler symptoms, our lives, livelihoods, and traffic patterns were, nonetheless, affected. The numerous consequences of COVID-19 on the health of our population and on the delivery of primary care services were substantial and will likely result in permanent changes to our approach to medical care and the relationships we have with our family doctors.

We all know that health insurance benefits and coverages greatly influence (and often fully dictate) our medical care. In the next chapter I will explore the many ways that major medical insurance involvement in the relationship between you and your doctor affects the quality of your care and access to it.

# 6

# The Effects of Insurance Involvement on Primary Care

Americans have a love-hate relationship with health insurance.

It is universally accepted that we all need health insurance, but selecting and paying for it is often frustrating and always complicated. Whether major medical insurance is offered to us through an employer or if we are shopping for it as an individual or for our family, there are invariably multiple plan options presented to us that include extensive and overwhelming details.

Since we aren't health insurance industry experts, we are faced with making a decision (on a deadline) without understanding all of the implications of our choice. And, although we feel like there is too much information and too many choices being presented to us, the choices are predefined by our employer, an insurance broker, or a health insurance marketplace "exchange" in accordance with the Patient Protection and Affordable Care Act (ACA) known as Obamacare.

This pick-a-card-any-card approach often finds us living with consequences that never occurred to us when we selected our insurance plan. Surprises may come up at the time you receive care but are most commonly realized long after the fact when the bill or Explanation of Benefits (EOB) arrives. Unexpected costs may be in the area of coverage (such as exclusions of coverage for various services) or in unexpected costs from deductibles or various categories of copayments.

As with most things in life, health insurance can be a mixed bag of good and bad. Major medical insurance is literally a life-saver when catastrophe strikes. It singularly allows Americans to expect high-quality, high-tech, modern care that is the envy of the world. When we require hospitalizations, surgeries, and chronic specialty care for serious medical conditions, we fully realize the value of having comprehensive health insurance.

We can receive care that hardly anyone would be able to afford without insurance. That's the good. The bad is in the many strings that are attached. Each insurance plan stipulates the conditions under which they will pay for services you receive. Medical services and products are only covered and reimbursed according to plan details, which determine where you receive care, who delivers the care, which doctors and facilities are in-network participating, which services (including types of visits, tests, and treatments) are allowed in network and out of network, what preventive and nonpreventive services are covered, your premiums, your deductibles, your copayments, your out-of-pocket limits, and what your doctors and other healthcare providers are paid and allowed to charge. Whew!

It is clear who is in charge of your healthcare. In this chapter, I briefly consider how and why health insurance began in the United States and how it has evolved. I also explore the six major challenges and disadvantages to health insurance involvement in the relationship between you and your primary care physician.

## The Development of Health Insurance

According to the Kaiser Family Foundation, 92% of all Americans have health insurance as do more than 99% of older Americans over the age of sixty-five. But it wasn't always that way.

One hundred years ago, medical care was inexpensive and, by today's standards, unsophisticated. Old Doc Brown would come to your house and deliver your baby in exchange for a chicken. The advances in medical science, diagnostic tools, as well as medical and surgical interventions since that time have been truly remarkable. Literally no one would want to return to the days before immunizations, antibiotics (and thousands of other medications for every condition imaginable), x-rays, MRIs, sterile surgery operating facilities, organ transplants, coronary artery bypass "open heart" and other life-saving surgeries, just to name a few.

Understandably, these substantial, near miraculous medical advancements come at a cost. The challenge ever since the early days of hospitals and modernization has been how to pay for the best care available.

In 1912, President Teddy Roosevelt endorsed the idea of social insurance that would have included health insurance. Others in government and the private sector attempted to advance the concept, but it wasn't until 1929 that the first prepaid health plan was introduced by the Baylor Hospital. It was an employer-sponsored plan that covered in-patient hospital services only and was offered to teachers in Dallas. The employer would pay the hospital a monthly fee (now considered a premium) to guarantee payment for the increasingly expensive technology and care being provided to their employees during hospital admissions. This Baylor plan is considered to be the forerunner of early nonprofit Blue Cross plans that would follow.

By 1930, physicians began to develop Blue Shield plans that would cover the costs of medical care that were provided by physicians. During World War II, employer-sponsored health insurance benefits grew dramatically due to federal wage control laws. Employers offered various expanded "fringe benefits" including comprehensive health insurance to attract new workers in a very tight labor market.

The explosion of employer-based health insurance during World War II led to the health insurance industry we have today. This industry includes both private companies and governmental programs offering insurance to employers as group plans and also directly to individuals and families.

The vast majority of individuals now choose their doctors and other health providers based on their providers' contractual participation with the covered member's health insurance carrier and plan. There are advantages and some significant disadvantages to this arrangement pertaining to people's relationships with their primary care physicians.

Health insurance protects participants from the full brunt of expensive and unexpected medical costs. This is an obvious benefit when people require hospitalization, surgery, or ongoing specialty care. Even with today's high deductibles and copayments, major medical insurance often significantly reduces out-of-pocket costs for individuals. This typically allows them to receive a high level of medical care they otherwise could not afford.

Half of the population of the US currently receives health insurance as an employee benefit through their employer who often pays all or a portion of the expense for medical insurance, making it feasible for most. Also, since participating providers bill patients' insurance directly and initially only collect estimated copayments and deductibles from patients, the timing of any portion of payment that is the patient's responsibility is delayed until claims are reviewed and discounted by the insurance carrier. Of course, these benefits represent the value that traditional health insurance provides to individuals. The benefits are most appreciated when individuals require unexpected and extremely high-dollar care.

Let's look at some significant disadvantages that will never be highlighted by insurance brokers or the benefits managers of employers.

## Six Major Disadvantages of Insurance Involvement in Primary Care

Virtually everyone understands the importance of major medical insurance as it relates to unexpected high-dollar care for severe injuries and significant medical conditions, but the value equation for health insurance is quite different when applied to coverage for primary care services.

The full potential cost for primary care services is neither expensive nor unpredictable. Routine and preventive care as well as the management of most acute illness and the majority of chronic disease processes by primary care physicians would be quite affordable for most Americans even if they had no health insurance at all. In fact, the involvement of health insurance in the relationship between patients and their primary care physicians introduces several major challenges and disadvantages. Here are the six primary areas of concern.

## 1. Non-Value-Added Middlemen

Insurance involvement makes primary care more expensive. It is estimated that as much as 40% of revenue paid to primary care physicians who participate with major health insurance goes to pay for administrative overhead, claims processing, insurance company profits, and the compensation of insurance brokers. This list of middlemen who mediate the interactions and care that you receive from your doctor do not actually add value to your quality of care or patient experience. They do add significant costs for your doctor, your employer, and ultimately you. In reality, inserting these middlemen between you and your doctor makes it more challenging for doctors to do their job.

Who pays your doctor? The answer makes all the difference to your access and customer service. So who pays your doctor? Your insurance company. Realistically, your doctor doesn't work for you. They work for your insurance company and spend a lot of time and money meeting their requirements. This insurance middleman increases your cost, kills convenience, and leads to poor health. Ask yourself how your care would be different if you and your physician weren't paying for these middlemen and your doctor wasn't working, in a manner of speaking, for your insurance company.

## 2. Volume-Based Care

When the delivery of healthcare services is adjudicated by insurance on a fee-for-service basis, your care is volume-based. Every service you receive, including lab work, other diagnostic tests, all treatments, examinations, discussions, and time with your doctor, only happens if these services are individually deemed covered and reimbursable by your insurance plan.

For physicians practicing under this (nearly universal) model, they are only paid if they are able to justify each individual service they render with codes (CPT procedure codes for specific ICD-10 diagnostic codes) and documentation that are acceptable to the insurance carrier. The amount your doctor is paid on a fee-for-service basis is locked and predetermined by a provider contract between your doctor and your insurance company.

Given the ever-increasing administrative and regulatory costs to operate a medical practice, the only way participating providers can sustain practice viability is by increasing the volume of patients they see. This dynamic of volume-based care is the main reason that primary care physicians are always rushed and access to care is limited, causing poor patient experience, worse health outcomes, and more downstream expense (as previously noted).

## 3. *Misaligned Incentives*

Why do doctors do what they do? Why do they require the visits that they do? Why do they order the tests that they order? The treatments? Make the referrals they make?

Medical doctors are regularly found to be among the most trustworthy professions (second only to nurses), but the vast majority of doctors practice in an environment that incentivizes them to ingratiate themselves by their ordering practices. Whether self-employed or working under employment agreements with medical practices that are most often owned by hospital systems, your doctor's take-home pay is largely determined by what the doctor's office bills. Just as volume-based care adds costs to the system, these misaligned incentives between you, your insurance company, and the ordering physician also add to the number of medical services that are performed.

Not only is physician compensation tied to the volume of patient visits that the doctor is able to accommodate into an overly busy schedule, but physicians may also be reimbursed directly or indirectly based on the number of ancillary services they order. These ancillary services include blood tests, other diagnostic tests, and treatments that they deliver in their office or through affiliated entities.

Hospitals, specifically, benefit greatly from the downstream medical care that is referred to their facilities by primary care physicians working directly for hospital-owned medical practices. This is the reason that their employment agreements typically compensate them based on their ordering practices. In this insurance-based fee-for-service system, even the most altruistic physicians may be ordering office visits, tests, treatments, and referrals that are questionable or altogether unnecessary. Your doctor's incentives are rarely ever actually in line with yours.

## *4. Noncovered Services*

There is another side to the coin. The ubiquitous volume-based, insurance-participating fee-for-service primary care practice model also may result in underdelivery of important medical services. Some important diagnostic and treatment services are deemed to be noncovered in certain situations. If your insurance carrier is unwilling to reimburse your doctor for a test or treatment that the doctor feels is important, the doctor will be less likely to recommend it. Physicians often know or can determine via a prior authorization process if your specific insurance plan will cover a test or treatment that they are considering.

If insurance is not willing to cover the procedure (or if it would be subject to a very high deductible and out-of-pocket expense to the patient), your doctor may choose not to recommend the procedure due to concern about your direct expense or fear that they may not collect payment at all. This is an example of the common reality that your doctor doesn't work for you but is beholden to your insurance company. They are conditioned that if insurance will not pay for a service, they "can't" order it. As you can imagine, this mindset has great potential to result in a compromise to the quality of patient care.

## *5. Hidden True Patient Costs*

Health insurance is a shell game. The true costs of healthcare services and the mark-up at each step in the system of delivery are well hidden. What does a service cost your doctor or the medical office to provide? What does it cost your employer? The insurance company? As a patient or covered member, you may never know.

Eventually, you will find out what it will cost you personally—but not until well after you have received the service. The complexity and multiple middlemen involved in health insurance pricing, repricing, and reimbursement currently make it nearly impossible for individuals to determine the real costs for medical services that they receive. Insurance premiums continue to skyrocket. Employers "share" an increasing amount and percentage of these premiums with their employees who are also left with higher out-of-pocket expenses from rising deductibles and copayments for all types of medical services.

In some cases, especially with services provided and ordered by primary care physicians, it is possible to identify true market-based cash prices. What would certain medical services (office visits, lab tests, x-rays, MRIs, prescription medications, for example) cost if you didn't have insurance at all?

It is fairly common for out-of-pocket payments for diagnostic and treatment services that are delivered by primary care physicians and filed with health insurance to exceed the market-based cash prices that could be paid (without insurance involvement) for the same services. The fact is, most patients never know it when their health insurance is delivering a penalty rather than a financial benefit. Historically, these disparities have not been disclosed by insurers. This long-standing industry practice leaves most patients overpaying for some medical services on a regular basis.

## *6. Deterrents to Care*

Health insurance is designed to limit how often and how quickly people go to the doctor. This is particularly true with primary care.

Copayments, deductibles, and other out-of-pocket expenses built into insurance plans have proven to deter patients from seeking timely and appropriate primary care. As health insurance has become increasingly expensive, deductibles and out-of-pocket costs have increased in order to keep premiums from rising even higher. When accessing most primary care services, patients pay first before their insurance kicks in. They are paying directly for more routine primary care services and become increasingly likely to postpone or avoid needed care.

According to a recent survey of 1,000 Americans conducted by 20|20 Research, 64% of Americans say they have avoided or delayed medical care in the last year due to expected costs. These costly insurance plan design mechanisms along with the other inefficiencies created by insurance involvement in your relationship with your doctor deter access to medical care that is otherwise uniquely available to people across our country.

## From My Practice

Back pain is one of the most common reasons people go to the doctor. Acute back pain is miserable and can stop you in your tracks. Severe low back pain with electric pain shooting down your leg is often suddenly debilitating.

My patient Willie couldn't get up off the floor. I spoke with him over the phone, and we agreed that he would call a friend to help him get into my office for an exam. He had had back pain in the past but nothing like this, and nothing with leg pain. His history and my examination of his back and neurological status made it seem likely that he had a herniated disk in his lumbar spine. I explained that, in most cases, a conservative approach of anti-inflammatory pills, muscle relaxants, stronger pain medication if needed, stretching exercises, continuing to cautiously move around, and time would usually get people back to normal, even when they have a herniated disk.

He asked about an MRI. Everybody wants to know what's going on. I let Willie know that there is typically no urgency to get an MRI unless we think he needs surgery immediately and that his insurance would be unlikely to pay for it, unless he was still having severe pain and leg symptoms after completing several weeks of physical therapy. He understood and went home with some pills.

The conservative approach didn't last long. Willie was miserable in spite of a prescription for hydrocodone, a narcotic pain medicine. After a couple of days, he was understandably insisting on doing something. Rather than going to the ER where they would probably give him more pain medication and send him home, we decided to pursue the MRI.

I tried. We submitted a request for prior authorization for the MRI of the lumbar spine. His insurance said it wasn't "medically necessary" (unless he did physical therapy first). Willie and I decided to do what we both thought was best and ordered an MRI. The MRI showed a severely herniated disk, which resulted in immediate referral to a neurosurgeon, followed by epidural injections that gave him fairly rapid pain relief.

Here are the morals of the story. The fact that Willie had major medical insurance did not help him. It affected our choice to delay a diagnostic test (MRI) that turned out to clearly prove the cause of his pain and set him up for timely and effective treatment. Insurance would have required him to have a prolonged course of physical therapy (at his expense) and ultimately pay the full cost of the MRI since he had not met his deductible. I was able to get him an MRI right away at a cash price of $260—dramatically less than the $1,005 he would have paid if an insurance claim was filed.

Our approach without insurance was better, faster, and cheaper. Willie was ultimately happy with his care and his doctor (me) but quite unhappy with his insurance.

## Get Insurance Out of Your Doctor's Office

Insurance involvement in the relationship between you and your primary care doctor doesn't provide the benefits that you thought it would.

Major medical insurance is essential in modern society in order for the vast majority of Americans to be able to receive and pay for high-tech, expensive, and unpredictable medical services. Insurance is intended and ideal for healthcare that is high cost and unexpected. It is a necessity when patients require surgeries and hospitalizations or experience major accidents and catastrophic medical diagnoses.

On the other hand, the whole of primary care medicine is neither expensive nor unpredictable, and placing its payment structure under the umbrella of a comprehensive medical plan only serves to increase cost and decrease care.

As we have seen, simply having health insurance does not guarantee quality primary care. In fact, inserting the middlemen required for a third party (insurance) to pay for some primary care services on your behalf disrupts the quality of your relationship with your doctor and greatly restricts your access to them.

In Part III of this book, I consider how people from coast to coast are sidestepping the traditional insurance-based fee-for-service primary care delivery model in favor of new alternatives that give them high-level access to fast and personal care from their primary care physicians.

# PART III

# HOW TO GET FAST, PERSONAL CARE FROM YOUR DOCTOR

# 7

# The Triple Aim of Healthcare

The delivery of primary care services in America needs to be improved.

It is clear that you need fast access to your personal doctor—a primary care physician who knows you, someone you can count on to answer your questions and provide care in a timely manner. It is equally clear that the majority of us find it frustrating when we attempt to get what we need—and can't.

In the following chapters you will learn that, while it is not typical in America today, you can receive a high level of care from physicians who practice in new and improved delivery systems and practice models that are highly affordable for nearly all Americans. These efficient models of primary care effectively accomplish the objectives that healthcare improvement organizations have been seeking for many years. First, let's consider the three primary objectives or aims of healthcare improvement.

Many healthcare organizations, institutes, medical societies, governmental initiatives, and agencies, as well as large numbers of other corporations, recognize the importance of fixing healthcare, including primary care. The Institute for Healthcare Improvement has introduced a widely adopted framework for approaching healthcare system improvement and optimization. In order for healthcare to be ideally effective, it must address three aspects of care: patient experience, health outcomes, and cost.

This triple aim is to achieve

1. Better care for individuals,
2. Better health for populations, and
3. Lower per capita costs.

To boil it down, the triple aim requires our healthcare delivery systems to move toward better, faster, and cheaper care. Better care speaks to improving the health or health outcomes for individuals and populations of people or communities. Faster care in terms of access, wait times, and customer service addresses improvements of the patient experience. Cheaper, less expensive care per capita is essential in order to increase the likelihood that a maximum number of people will be able to avail themselves of the improved better and faster care.

Conventional wisdom states that it is possible to choose any two of these elements but that simultaneously achieving the improvement of all three is unlikely or impossible. However, improvement of all three components is exactly what our system requires.

As it relates to the care of individuals, high-level access to a personal primary care physician and the efficient delivery of primary care services presents an enormous opportunity to accomplish all three objectives of the triple aim.

I established in Part I of this book that primary care physician relationships are potentially the most efficient and logical way for people to get answers to their questions and to receive care for the majority of their medical conditions. Primary care is also widely recognized as being crucial to the execution of optimal preventive care, individual adoption of healthy lifestyle, and the early detection of disease. In many respects primary care can and should serve as the foundation and initial point of care for the entire healthcare system.

## 1. Better Care

The first leg of the triple aim is to actually improve patient care. For individuals, their perception of better primary care is closely tied to the experience they have when interacting with their doctor and the doctor's office staff. As discussed in chapter 4, the patient experience encompasses both service quality and other aspects of care that patients value highly such as receiving timely appointments, gaining easy access to information, and having good communication both via telephone and electronic means as well as verbally when physically present in the doctor's office.

Superior patient experience consists of high-quality medical care and also high-quality customer service. Patient satisfaction requires that primary care physicians and their delivery systems provide excellent access to the physician who knows the patient best. Timely access and adequate amounts of time with the doctor improve diagnostic accuracy, patient comprehension about their condition, trust in their physician, and compliance with recommended treatments. All of this improves patients' clinical outcomes.

Research on patient satisfaction and doctor-patient relationship reveals that satisfaction with care is directly related to the amount of time that patients spend face-to-face with their doctor in discussion of their condition, treatment effects, health education, and also on physical examination. In addition to time and their doctor's communication skills, patients also associate excellent care with the ability to receive same-day appointments with their personal physician, minimal waiting time in the doctor's office, unhurried visits, and the ability to quickly and directly communicate with their doctor when not in the office (via phone, text, email, and video chat).

Significant effort has been put forth over the past twenty years by large healthcare entities and other industry participants to enhance the patient experience across entire healthcare systems. Much of these efforts have been focused on communication. Tools and organizations have been developed to assist patients in better navigating the healthcare system, to help providers communicate with each other and their patients, to integrate and coordinate disparate healthcare entities, and to hold each component accountable to quality-of-care measures.

Electronic medical records (EMR) or electronic health records (EHR) organize information and allow for more efficient billing, scheduling, and sharing of health information among providers and also between patients and their doctors.

Managed Care Organizations (MCOs) refer to entities that seek to save money on healthcare while providing better services for patients. They exist in three main categories: Health Maintenance Organizations (HMOs), Preferred Provider Organizations (PPOs), and Point of Service plans with numerous iterations and areas of focus. Examples of these include Independent Physician or Practice Associations (IPAs), Integrated Delivery Organizations, Physician Practice Management Companies, Group Purchasing Organizations, Integrated Delivery Systems, Physician-Hospital Organizations, Management Services Organizations, and Accountable Care Organizations. Accountable Care Organizations (ACOs) are groups of doctors, hospitals, and other healthcare providers who organize voluntarily to attempt to more efficiently coordinate the care of Medicare beneficiaries and patients with private insurance. Descriptions and discussions of the myriad of other MCOs is beyond the scope of this chapter.

Another important initiative to improve the care, experience, and satisfaction of patients is to ask them for their feedback. Healthcare organizations are continuously attempting to gather information from patients through patient satisfaction surveys and other means to track the impact of their systemwide changes on quality improvement measures or outcomes. Of course, implementing changes suggested by patient surveys as well as delivery system improvements realized through the formation of various Managed Care Organizations happen exceedingly slowly and at great expense. This process also introduces layers of middlemen between the respondents to surveys and the doctors and staff who are rendering care. The providers in this case are unlikely to feel directly accountable to this feedback from their customers.

It is my belief and experience that many of the most impactful quality improvement measures that enhance patient care and experience are identified and implemented on the frontlines of new value-based primary care practices that I discuss in the following chapters.

## 2. Better Health

The second goal of the triple aim recognizes that patient experience and customer satisfaction are dependent on results or clinical outcomes. The ultimate goal of the practice of medicine is to keep people healthy and improve their quality and longevity of life—to prevent disease, illness, and injury.

While the focus of this element within the triple aim, as defined by the Institute for Healthcare Improvement, is on improving population health, let's consider the search for better health from the perspective of the individual. Your health: getting healthy and staying healthy, when begun early, is largely the domain of preventive medicine. Currently in the United States, compliance with preventive measures that are known to be beneficial and life-prolonging is at disappointingly low levels. In each of the categories of preventive medicine, there is much room for improvement.

Preventive health measures are generally categorized in the following four groups: primordial, primary, secondary, and tertiary.

- **Primordial** prevention is the reduction of risk factors that are targeted toward entire populations via improving social and environmental conditions. Examples of primordial prevention are improved access to healthy foods within a community, building public walking paths to encourage exercise, or increasing the taxes on cigarettes to deter smoking.

- **Primary** prevention is focused on preventing a disease from ever occurring in an individual. Examples of primary prevention would be immunizations to prevent COVID-19 and multiple other infectious diseases, smoking cessation programs to prevent the development of lung cancer, emphysema, and cardiovascular disease, or improving dietary habits before medical conditions like obesity, diabetes, high cholesterol, and hypertension have a chance to develop.

- **Secondary** prevention is screening to identify diseases in their earliest stages before any signs or symptoms develop. Many serious medical conditions are dangerously far advanced by the time they cause symptoms. Cancers of the lung, prostate, breast, or colon as well as atherosclerotic cardiovascular disease that causes heart attacks and strokes are the most common causes of death in the US and most often have poor outcomes if they aren't detected prior to the development of symptoms. Examples of secondary prevention are blood pressure screening, mammography for early detection of breast cancer, screening colonoscopy for early detection of colon cancer, and Pap smear tests for early detection of cervical cancer.

- **Tertiary** prevention aims to reduce the severity and effects of a disease or its recurrence once it is diagnosed and symptomatic in an individual. Examples of tertiary prevention are cardiac rehabilitation after a heart attack (including dietary improvements, weight loss, and aggressive treatment of cholesterol, blood pressure, and diabetes), physical or occupational therapy after a stroke, diabetic foot care, and chemotherapy after a cancer diagnosis.

When structured and utilized appropriately, primary care is uniquely situated to address each of these phases of prevention. Primary care physicians can provide a broad range of health education, disease detection, and disease management services, which are proven to favorably affect health outcomes. When in a long-term trusting relationship with their patients, primary care physicians also provide consistent recurrent encouragement and accountability with their patients to adopt and maintain healthy lifestyles and follow through with periodic preventive screenings as recommended.

One of the main functions of primary care physicians is to provide each one of these key preventive medicine components that have been shown to deliver the greatest impact on long-term health:

- Health risk identification
- Timely preventive screenings
- Early detection of disease
- Lifestyle modification counseling
- Efficient disease management over time

To prevent disease, maintain optimal health, and maximize quality health-years, primary care physicians must work with their patients to focus on all of these key components that contribute to effect preventive medicine services. Improvements in these areas may be implemented through large system accountability and also at the individual physician practice level.

## 3. Lower Costs

The final objective of the triple aim is to make healthcare services more affordable. The US healthcare system is the most expensive in the world with total healthcare costs of nearly 18% of gross domestic product (GDP), with growth in personal healthcare spending projected to average 5.5% annually through 2026. A study published in *JAMA* in 2019 estimated the cost of waste in the US healthcare system between $760 billion and $935 billion each year, which is about 25% of total healthcare spending. The largest source of waste was believed to be administrative costs squandering a full $266 billion per year.

The next most wasteful category was found to be noncompetitive and nontransparent pricing to the tune of $241 billion per year. In large multi-entity and highly regulated healthcare systems, there are plenty of ideas about how to address cost and waste, but implementation of effective initiatives that actually move the needle have been elusive.

Better access to primary care services has the potential to be a significant contributor to bringing down overall healthcare costs. It can also reduce administrative waste and address many of the issues we have with the pricing of healthcare services. Increased utilization of primary care physician services has been shown to decrease overall healthcare costs by decreasing the need for expensive downstream emergency and specialty care. Specialty care is predictably overutilized when access to primary care is restricted or in short supply.

When people can't reach their primary care doctor right away, they seek answers and treatment from urgent care or hospital emergency departments or schedule appointments directly with specialists.

The beneficial effect of primary care on preventive health and disease management as well as the inherent affordability of primary care compared with specialty care are felt to be the reasons for this lowering of costs. According to a national study of 13,270 adults, after adjustment for demographics, health insurance status, reported diagnoses, health perceptions, and smoking status, respondents who reported using a primary care physician had 33% lower annual adjusted healthcare expenditures and lower adjusted mortality than those who had no identified physicians or those who used specialist physicians exclusively.

In the trenches of primary care, the doctors' experience, judgment, and knowledge of the healthcare system may provide immediate and significant cost savings to their patients. The more conditions that are diagnosed and treated by the primary care physician, the fewer tests are ordered, fewer hospitalizations occur, and not as many surgeries are performed.

In addition, issues with price variations and price transparency may be reduced or eliminated by primary care doctors. Physicians practicing in new value-based models are more likely to have the time and ability to shop for the best prices for their patients on lab tests, imaging (x-rays, CT scans, MRIs) and make prescription medication choices that are highly affordable to their patients. Finally, many of the reasons for administrative waste are curtailed or eliminated altogether in the new value-based primary care delivery models that will be covered in the next chapter.

## From My Practice

A longtime patient of mine recently referred his brother, Tony, to my practice. Tony is a young (thirty-one-year-old) healthy guy who never thought he needed a doctor—until he did. He got in a car wreck on a Thursday night. It was more than a fender bender, and his neck was getting stiff at the scene of the accident, but he really didn't want to go to the ER.

By the next morning his neck really hurt. He had a splitting headache and felt a little lightheaded. He needed a doctor but didn't know one that he could call. He hadn't had a regular doctor since his mom took him to the pediatrician as a teen. Since he was in pain, he decided he needed to see a doctor somewhere. Instead of the ER, he went to a walk-in urgent care clinic expecting that it would be faster and cheaper. His insurance would cover it, right?

Tony arrived at the urgent care just after noon on Friday and was surprised by a busy waiting room. He waited just under an hour before he was taken back to see the doctor (actually a nurse practitioner). After a few questions and a five-minute exam, he was told he would need x-rays of his neck and a CT scan of his brain. Since the urgent care was owned by the hospital, they had those imaging tests available in the same building. He waited another forty minutes.

After the tests were completed and images reviewed by one of the urgent care doctors, he was told they looked fine and he could go home and take ibuprofen for the pain. They would let him know within a couple of days if the radiologist who would review the tests saw anything that the urgent care doctor might have missed. Tony was also told to go see a neurologist if his headaches didn't go away in a few days.

Oh, he was at a facility that was participating with his insurance plan, and the services were considered covered. But he didn't remember that his insurance was a High Deductible Health Plan (HDHP) with a $2,000 deductible and, since he never went to the doctor, it hadn't been touched. That meant that

Tony would be responsible for the entire bill: $150 for the nurse practitioner visit, $142 for the cervical spine x-rays, and $720 for the CT scan. His trip to urgent care, which resulted only in a recommendation to take ibuprofen, cost him about three hours and over $1,000 out of his pocket. That's expensive ibuprofen!

Although he had health insurance, Tony didn't have a doctor. Without fast access to a personal primary care physician, his single trip to urgent care failed on all three of the triple aim objectives. It wasn't excellent care or a satisfying patient experience, and it certainly wasn't cost effective.

When I saw Tony for the first time and he told me about this experience, I shared with him how this medical need would have been taken care of quite differently if he had been a patient in my practice a little sooner. Tony now has my direct mobile phone number. He could have called me from the scene of the accident and asked if I felt he needed to go to the ER immediately. From his description, he would not.

I would have coached him for what red flags to be on the lookout for, and, when he awakened on Friday with increased symptoms, I would have asked him to come to my office right away to be examined. Based on his examination, he may have needed x-rays of his cervical spine but certainly would not have needed a CT scan of his head. His x-rays would have cost him $46, been read by a radiologist immediately, and he would have had no additional charge for my visit or examination.

Because he is now in a membership-based practice, he has unrestricted access to his doctor for a flat monthly fee (in his case $55). His care with a primary care physician in a value-based practice is better, faster, and cheaper. His out-of-pocket cost for that one visit to the urgent care would have paid for nearly two years of unlimited office visits, phone calls, and texts for every question and problem he might have.

## Better, Faster, Cheaper

Many aspects of healthcare in America need improvement. Healthcare in the US is generally the best in the world and the most expensive. We have a complex system that will forever need to be revised, updated, and made more efficient. The triple aim of improving the quality of care (patient experience), health outcomes (individual and population health), and cost effectiveness (per capita cost) will define our focus in the foreseeable future.

Simply carrying health insurance coverage doesn't guarantee you excellence in any of these areas. Better access to primary care services in conjunction with a personal primary care physician who knows you and is always available, absolutely does. Such an arrangement addresses all aspects of the triple aim for the majority of medical needs that most of us will have in a given year.

I have hinted at a new and improved approach to achieving high-level access to your primary care physician. In the next chapter, I explore the concepts of value-based care and Direct Primary Care. I will compare and contrast these models with the traditional volume-based standard that you may have experienced up until now, which often produces a frustrating lack of access to your doctor.

# 8

# Value-Based Care and Direct Primary Care (DPC)

So far, I have explored mostly intuitive arguments for why you need a doctor and why finding one that will provide what you know you need has been so difficult. I have described the current state of primary care and the reasons why the traditional volume-based fee-for-service third-party-insurance-mediated model that is ubiquitous across our country fails to provide adequate access to primary care physicians.

We've all seen that the results of this current system are delayed care, poor health outcomes, higher overall costs, and frustrated patients. Now it's time to consider a better approach: a primary care delivery model that is currently providing hundreds of thousands of Americans with affordable, high-level access to their personal primary care physician.

Fortunately for Americans today, forward-thinking providers and insurers are recognizing the problems with volume-based care and are gravitating toward value-based delivery models. In various forms, the concept of value-based payment models is to compensate physicians, physician practices, and other healthcare entities for favorable outcomes instead of how many times they turn the turnstile (in other words, the volume and types of billing codes filed to insurance).

In some iterations, value-based care harkens to the days of Health Maintenance Organizations (HMOs) of the 1970s through the 1990s when many Managed Care Organizations entered into capitated payment arrangements with contracted physicians. They were paid a fixed payment per patient (member) per month (PMPM) in attempts to eliminate inadvertent physician incentives to inappropriately overutilize tests and treatments. However, the alternative incentive that these arrangements created was to limit utilization of necessary services and deny access to care. Spending was cut, but at the expense of quality patient care. Compensation addressed cost but did not improve health outcomes or patient experience.

Unlike these dinosaur arrangements of the past, the value-based models currently in practice focus on desired outcomes in all three aspects of the triple aim.

This chapter briefly describes several value-based delivery models that have been introduced by the Centers for Medicare & Medicaid Services (CMS) and numerous private health insurance carriers. These models will be compared and contrasted. I will then describe in more detail a unique independent "grassroots" movement of private physicians practicing in a very efficient direct-to-consumer "insurance-free" value-based primary care reimbursement model known as Direct Primary Care (DPC).

## Insurance-Driven Value-Based Models

Healthcare costs are out of control and volume-based insurance reimbursement models are felt to be contributing to the problem. Medicare and most major private medical insurance carriers have begun testing and transitioning to reimbursement models that pay for healthcare services based on the *quality* of care instead of the *quantity* of services provided. These quality-based or value-based reimbursement models reward healthcare providers for providing the best care possible as efficiently as possible. They also have the effect of shifting some amount of financial risk from the insurance carrier to the healthcare provider.

Physicians, hospitals, and other providers must assume the risk that they will be able to improve the level of care and health outcomes while simultaneously cutting the costs to deliver care. With the aforementioned pressures on primary care practices, assuming risk of reimbursement for services performed is not an easy sell for smaller physician-owned practices but is being adopted by larger primary care practices and many that are owned by hospitals.

Since Medicare is by far the largest health insurance payer in the US and is therefore a very influential buyer of healthcare services, it has led the way in developing programs that encourage healthcare providers to coordinate care and assume risk of outcomes in these value-based reimbursement models. The Affordable Care Act and the Centers for Medicare & Medicaid Services (CMS) encouraged the formation of Accountable Care Organizations (ACOs) consisting of various healthcare providers that join together to coordinate care and enter into contracts with Medicare and commercial insurance companies.

Many ACOs are organized by large hospital systems that enter into these alternate payment arrangements with public and private payers. As of January 2021, providers had formed 477 ACOs across the country that serve more than 10.7 million Medicare beneficiaries and several hundred additional ACOs contracting with Medicaid and private insurance companies. CMS has also recently launched Primary Care First, a new program that will provide primary care services to Medicare and Medicaid recipients under a value-based reimbursement model with physician practices.

In another approach to value-based care, some private insurance carriers and captive health plans are offering access to primary care clinics with little or no fee-for-service costs to the participants. Insurance carriers have employed primary care physicians and midlevel providers at dedicated insurance-owned clinics that provide a full range of primary care services to members of the insurance plan. Private payers are hopeful that expanded access to primary care services, sometimes during extended office hours, with no office visit or lab charges to the patient will encourage the use of these clinics and consequently limit care provided through other medical providers, thus shrinking insurance claims, minimizing downstream specialty care, and lowering cost.

While these approaches seem to mitigate some of the limitations of traditional volume-based primary care, many of the disadvantages of our existing primary care delivery approach that were enumerated previously still remain. Members of these plans are only able to access care when these clinics are open. They may see a different provider each time they require care, and, in the event that their employer no longer offers a plan with access to these primary care clinics, they are forced to start over with a new primary care physician.

Maybe the greatest limitation to these value-based care models is the fact that the reimbursement and therefore the care are still being driven by the insurance carrier, rather than by the patient and their personal physician.

## Direct Primary Care

The value-based care delivery model that is growing rapidly and organically among practicing primary care physicians across America is known as Direct Primary Care (DPC). Direct Primary Care is a membership-based primary care payment model in which patients (or their employers or health plans) pay a flat monthly/periodic fee directly to the DPC physician practice in exchange for unrestricted access to their personal physician.

This periodic fee is typically under $100 per month and entitles the member to high-level access to all or most acute care, disease management, and preventive services available at the primary care practice. These fees are not filed to health insurance plans and are typically not reimbursed by them. The three characteristics that generally define DPC practices are that DPC practices

- Charge a periodic fee,
- Do not bill any third parties (insurance) on a fee-for-service basis, and
- Per-visit charges (if any) must be less than the monthly membership fee.

A provision in the Affordable Care Act, championed by the DPC Coalition, defines DPC as an innovative care delivery model "allowing consumers to gain access to an affordable and reliable source of primary services." Over thirty states have subsequently passed laws or regulations establishing DPC as a medical service regulated by state boards of medicine outside of third-party insurance reimbursement. These key policy changes allow employers to offer DPC a valuable health benefit, which is not considered a health plan under state insurance regulations.

DPC is not concierge medicine. The characteristics of DPC practices are in contrast with concierge practices, which generally are much more expensive than $100 per month and also bill insurance for each service rendered, in addition to charging members a retainer or access fee.

The first DPC practice to adopt this model began in Seattle in 1997, one year after the first concierge medicine practice was established. Seattle Medical Associates was converted to a DPC practice by Garrison Bliss, MD, and charged $65 per month while MD$^2$, the first known concierge practice, charged an annual retainer fee of $13,200 to $20,000 per family. Parenthetically, by the time my medical practice (ProPartners Healthcare in metro Kansas City) transitioned to the DPC model in 2013, there were only about fifty such practices in the country. Today, there are about 1,500 independent physician practices in forty-eight states and the District of Columbia that provide services under this model.

## *Scope of Services*

DPC is largely a cottage industry that has been established and is being expanded by entrepreneurial primary care physicians in solo and small group physician-owned practices across the US. Due to this grassroots development, there are variations in practice design and services. In most cases, DPC practices offer high-level 24/7 access to a personal physician via phone, email, text messaging, same-day appointments for general medical care, extended office visits, virtual visits via phone or video, and often a variety of other primary care services (preventive care, in-office procedures, minor surgeries, EKG, spirometry, vision and hearing screening, among others) all included for a flat monthly fee.

There are typically no office visit charges or any additional costs for the physician's time, regardless of how often the patient requires care. Other ancillary services offered in DPC offices are either free or offered at cost such as lab tests, immunizations, and prescription medications. DPC practices may also negotiate significantly discounted cash prices for their members with area imaging centers (x-ray, ultrasound, CT scan, MRI) and other providers (physician specialists, physical therapists, dietitians, for example) and pass the savings on to their members at wholesale prices.

## *Value Proposition*

The affordable and high-level access to a personal physician that is promised by the DPC value-based care model is made possible largely due to the elimination of the insurance middleman. The cost to deliver primary care drops significantly when this non-value-added intermediary is removed. The physician and medical practice are able to eliminate all of the time and expenses associated with filing and refiling insurance claims, negotiating disputed claims, balance billing patients, adjusting off unpaid charges, and satisfying the insurance carriers' complex requirements for documentation and coding in order to be reimbursed.

The immediate result of this simplification is that DPC physicians are able to reduce the number of patients they care for dramatically compared with the patient panel that almost every insurance-participating (volume-based) physician carries, freeing up a significant amount of time to be available to their patient members. This allows them to be highly accessible to their patients by phone, text, or same-day appointment.

Under the DPC model, physicians work directly for their patients rather than their patients' insurance companies and are directly accountable to patients for all decisions and costs related to their medical care. This simplified direct-to-consumer model eliminates the enormous administrative load that is inherent in any reimbursement arrangement being adjudicated by a third-party payer.

Even with new value-based payment contracts offered by insurance companies and Medicare/Medicaid, the cumulative costs for the organizations involved to calculate and determine payment to providers is substantial. DPC eliminates these expenses. If a patient determines that the value of having enhanced access, availability, and time with their personal primary care doctor is worth the monthly membership fee, they stay with the DPC practice. If not, they don't. The accountability is immediate, and the value is in the eye of the customer—who is also the payer!

## Benefits of DPC

Value-based Direct Primary Care provides several key benefits that volume-based insurance-brokered traditional primary care cannot consistently deliver.

## *Time and Access*

Direct Primary Care physicians get paid to be available. Patients pay for the peace of mind that their personal doctor will be there when they need them. As previously described, eliminating insurance from the primary care equation decreases the cost of care. This reduction in overhead allows DPC physicians to limit their patient panels to an average of 400 to 800 total patients—less than a third of typical insurance-based primary care physicians who are almost always responsible for more than 2,000 patients. This effectively triples the amount of time DPC physicians have available for each of their patients.

The DPC membership fee guarantees patients that their doctor will be available when needed via quick responses to phone calls, emails, and texts, same-day/next-day appointments, extended length visits, and an unrestricted number of doctor visits. Since each DPC physician is caring for a significantly reduced number of patients, appointments are not rushed, so the doctor has the time to listen and get to know and build a relationship with each patient.

In addition to investing more time in diagnosis and explanation of recommendations, the DPC physician is able to be proactive in following up with each patient and recalling them for periodic disease management, health screening tests, and preventive care. Finally, this additional time devoted to each patient allows the physician to become an advocate and adviser to help their patients to efficiently and cost-effectively navigate a complex American healthcare system.

## *Aligned Incentives*

Another benefit of not having health insurance involved in the relationship between primary care physicians and patients is that it is always clear who the doctor works for. A physician who is paid a flat membership fee by their patients is directly and solely accountable to their patients and is highly motivated to maximize the patients' health, customer service, and satisfaction. The doctor's incentive is to maintain high patient satisfaction, which is directly related to fast response times to calls, minimal waiting in the doctor's office, and better communication during visits and when the patient is not in the office.

Not only are incentives aligned around service quality, but DPC arrangements typically offer at-cost pricing on labs and other in-office testing so there is no incentive for a DPC doctor to ever order a test that the doctor does not believe is absolutely necessary. Doctor and patient are also aligned to avoid unnecessary trips to the doctor's office and unnecessary referrals as the DPC practice is never compensated on a fee-for-service basis for conducting more office visits or referring a patient for care elsewhere.

## *Downstream Care and Costs*

High-level timely access to Direct Primary Care has been shown to decrease the need for downstream emergency and specialty care, which results in a significant savings in overall healthcare costs. While few studies in the literature have analyzed savings from DPC, a recent two-year review of healthcare claims data on 3,088 patients receiving care under the DPC model demonstrated a 20% decrease in overall healthcare costs while also improving patient outcomes and satisfaction with care.

Specifically, this study demonstrated a decrease in ER visits (65% reduction), hospitalization days (43% reduction), specialist visits (66% reduction), MRI and CT scans (63% reduction), and surgeries (82% reduction) while simultaneously decreasing patients' total out-of-pocket healthcare expenses.

Another two-year literature review released in May 2020 by the DPC Coalition, American Academy of Family Physicians, Milliman, and the Society of Actuaries also concluded that the physician access delivered by Direct Primary Care and similar practice models shows lower overall healthcare claims costs, fewer hospitalizations, and lower emergency department utilization rates.

Finally, securing guaranteed access to their personal primary care physician through a DPC arrangement decreases the likelihood that members will have significant out-of-pocket expenses or meet their deductible on a routine basis. This enhanced access allows many DPC members to choose less expensive health insurance plans with higher deductibles and/or less coverage for primary care visits. In some instances, patients save as much in insurance premiums as they pay for DPC services. The details of how to choose health insurance plans that complement Direct Primary Care are elaborated in chapter 10.

## *Benefits for Employers*

Just as the efficiencies generated by Direct Primary Care benefit individuals wishing to secure access to quality primary care, there are several benefits to employers for sponsoring DPC memberships for their employees. There is evidence that providing DPC memberships to employees as the front end to major medical insurance benefits decreases overall health benefits costs to employers and employees by as much as 20% through all of the mechanisms covered previously.

With guaranteed access to primary care through an independent physician group, employers are free to select the insurance carrier, plan, and type of coverage that best complements the DPC benefit. This may mean avoiding being overinsured by obtaining a plan that carves out the primary care services already included in DPC membership, offering less expensive high-deductible plans, and/or choosing a partially level-funded or fully self-funded plan. Each of these options is likely to be less costly to the company and well-received by employees, especially in conjunction with the premium benefit of Direct Primary Care.

In the inevitable event that the major medical insurance carrier or plans change, the DPC relationship may be retained, ensuring that all employees may "keep their doctor" and maintain seamless continuity of their primary care. Further, efficient access and virtual care decrease absenteeism and time away from work due to otherwise lengthy wait times inherent in traditional volume-based practices. Finally, DPC membership improves employee loyalty and is perceived by employees as a premium benefit.

## From My Practice

Earlier in the section, I explained the triple aim of healthcare quality improvement and how it applies to primary care. As it turns out, several people in the healthcare reform world have recommended adding additional aims to grow the triple aim to a quadruple aim.

The aim that resonates with me as being most beneficial to patients and also healthcare providers (like myself) was described by Dave Chase and advanced by his organization, Health Rosetta, in 2015. It is the goal of improving the work life of healthcare providers, including clinicians and staff. This aim recognizes the widespread dissatisfaction and burnout of primary care physicians and the consequence that Chase describes like this: "Burnout is associated with lower patient satisfaction, reduced health outcomes, and it may increase costs. Burnout thus imperils the Triple Aim."

Let me tell you about my pursuit of the quadruple aim of healthcare improvement in my medical practice. ProPartners Healthcare was a unique primary care practice from the beginning. I founded the practice four days before 9/11 (that's right, the 2001 attack on the World Trade Center, Pentagon, and the third target occurred four days into my new business). We began as a primary care practice just for men and grew quickly to a practice with three full-time physicians and a physician's assistant in a busy insurance-participating fee-for-service practice with as many as 11,000 patients.

For several years, each physician was responsible for over 3,000 patients and saw more than twenty-five patients per day in the office. While we always tried to do "today's work today," our patients frequently wished they had faster access to their doctor or that we had more time to spend with them during their visits. In this volume-based model, it would never be possible—and the other doctors, staff, and I were definitely in burnout mode.

In early 2013, my partners heard about a new kind of membership-based medical practice model: Direct Primary Care. There weren't any DPC practices in the Kansas City area at the time, but we arranged a meeting with a DPC physician in Wichita who graciously told us about his early experience in doing away with health insurance contracts and enrolling patients who would pay him a monthly fee for unrestricted access to his care.

While we were nervous about how many of our patients would choose to stay when we told them we would no longer participate with their insurance plans, we were confident that this change would allow us to deliver better quality care, be more accessible to the patients who chose to stay, would likely save them money, and keep us sane.

We began a transition to the DPC model in the fall of 2013 and were practicing insurance-free membership-based care exclusively by early 2014. Soon after, we added a (female) family medicine physician and expanded into a DPC family practice.

Here's what happened. We didn't fire any patients or staff, but our number of patients, those who decided to stick with us, and our number of staff dropped significantly. Our billing staff moved on and were not replaced. The number of phones, computers, equipment, and square footage that the practice required went down along with our total expenses. Our average number of patient appointments for each physician per day dropped to about ten (from twenty-five), and half of those were virtual visits via phone or video chat. Each doctor's panel was now in the 400 to 700 patient range, our availability to our patients skyrocketed, and our stress levels plummeted.

Initially, about 15% of our patients became members, but over time, an interesting thing happened. We have had numerous past patients return to our practice with similar stories. Basically, they said, "Now I get it," and "I didn't know how good I had it." Many told us they couldn't find a doctor that could get them in quickly for an appointment, could never talk with them via phone, and they were always frustrated with the office staff and lack of return calls. They experienced the frustrations of volume-based primary care and decided that the benefits of Direct Primary Care that we promised them were worth the modest monthly fee. They quickly became believers in DPC and even advocates of the practice, referring family and friends on a regular basis.

## The Future of Healthcare Is Paying for Value

The quality of healthcare including primary care will improve to the degree that delivery systems focus on and reward the proper outcomes and results. Moving away from fee-for-service payment structures, which incentivize quantity over quality, and toward results-driven quality measures and value-based care as the basis for compensating providers is already under way.

The American healthcare industry, which consists of nearly 800,000 companies and generates over $1 trillion per year in direct patient care revenue, is complicated, cumbersome, slow, overregulated, and administratively bloated. The large players in the industry including regional and local hospital systems and governmental and private third-party payers are necessary to one degree or another for emergency care, specialty care, hospitalizations, and surgeries but add unnecessary bureaucracy and significant expense to the delivery of primary care services.

Fortunately, you can now consistently receive fast and personal care from a doctor who knows you and will remain your primary physician regardless of changes in your health insurance coverage. Direct Primary Care physicians' motives and incentives are aligned with yours. They are highly motivated to keep you happy and healthy since they work directly for you. You are paying them to always be available when you need them and to take the time to listen to you and to educate you about your care. You can also expect to save money by having a doctor who is "outside the system" as an advocate in your care.

In the next chapter I cover what to look for when selecting a new primary care physician and where you can locate a doctor who delivers medical care in a value-based DPC practice near you.

# 9

# How to Select and Establish Care with a Primary Care Physician

Do you have a doctor?

Even if you historically never go to the doctor, you need one. Do you have a personal primary care physician who knows you and will always be available when you need them? A relationship with a trusted primary care physician over time is crucial to every individual's health and well-being. Given the current state of primary care in post-pandemic America, many people either do not have a primary care physician or are dissatisfied with the lack of timely access to care and the hurried nature of their doctor's practice.

When you are inevitably faced with an immediate need or just realize that you would benefit from a long-term professional relationship with a doctor, how will you go about finding the right one? Hopefully, by now, you will be looking for more than just a random name picked from a list of participating providers on your insurance company's website.

In this chapter, I recommend and advise you to go through a process that includes judging various aspects of care and prioritizing what is most important to you. Too many people are quick to choose a doctor without first considering these factors. They stumble into a habit of going to a particular doctor's office without ever asking if it was the best choice.

I review six main factors you should consider as you locate and select a physician that is most likely to be a fit as a long-term primary care physician for you. I help you identify primary care physicians and practices that are likely to meet high expectations of care and service.

While it shouldn't be the sole or even primary determining factor, the major medical health insurance that you have must be considered when choosing a doctor. The other important elements in the selection process include physician credentials, online and other reviews, personal referrals and recommendations, the availability and ease of access to the doctor and his or her staff, the breadth of services that are offered in the medical practice, the location of the office or offices, your ability to quickly build a personal relationship, comfort, and rapport with the doctor, and the overall value you expect to receive from the relationship.

## Insurance Participation

Ever since employer-sponsored group medical plans became the norm decades ago and Preferred Provider Organizations (PPOs) and Health Maintenance Organizations (HMOs) began contracting with physicians, enrollees in these plans have been encouraged (or forced) to choose their doctors from their network of participating providers. Significant financial incentives are built into most health insurance plans that compel subscribers to stay in network for all of their care. Due to these plan structures, if employees want to take advantage of the employee benefit of health insurance, the primary if not sole factor that many people consider in choosing a doctor is their participation with the health insurance plan.

Selecting a primary care physician who is a participating provider in network with your insurance plan has the advantage of offsetting the costs of care from that doctor but has no effect on your costs for the types of medical care that can really get expensive. As long as the specialists, hospitals, and other healthcare providers that your primary care doctor refers you to for surgeries and hospitalizations are participating with your insurance, these costly services will be covered. This realization should encourage people who are looking for a primary care physician to consider other factors in choosing their doctor. They should ask many questions in addition to "Do you take my insurance?"

While the knee-jerk response from people looking for a doctor is still to simply pick from a list of participating providers supplied by their health plan, a physician's inclusion as an in-network provider does not guarantee quality care, an acceptable patient experience, or even reasonable out-of-pocket costs. Patient satisfaction with care is much more closely related to each of the determining factors enumerated next than it is with insurance participation of the doctor. Selecting a physician solely on the basis of insurance participation frequently leads to frustration with the quality of care and lack of responsive service.

Remember, it is very likely that your health plan is structured to pay contracted doctors on a fee-for-service basis, which creates the volume-driven misaligned incentive issues that I have covered in Part II of this book. It is advisable to avoid basing the selection of this important health provider on a list of physicians determined by your employer. These doctors are practicing in a volume-based fee-for-service system that makes it difficult for any of them to have the time to be available when you need them.

Along with all of the other determining factors discussed next, please consider the possibility that the best primary care physician for you, as well as the most cost-effective care, may be found outside of your health insurance network.

## Credentials, Reviews, and Personal Referrals

Do you know the background and credentials of your doctor? Where did they train? Where have they lived and practiced? What do other people have to say about them? Do you know anyone who has recommended them?

Educational and licensing credentials as well as patient reviews and personal referrals are all important elements to research when looking for a primary care physician. The education and training of a primary care physician is obviously important. You should be able to find a great deal of this information online, if you know where to look. Fortunately, state licensure, state boards of healing arts, and specialty boards ensure a level of safety, competency, and expertise for all physicians, and any legal or malpractice issues are published publicly by state boards.

Patients should do a quick check with their state medical board for these types of issues for any physician they are considering. Physicians' listings with state boards will include the doctor's age, license status (active), license number, specialty, address and phone number, medical school and graduation date as well as their status with continuing medical education. A listing of all state medical boards with their contact information may be found at the Federation of State Medical Boards website: www.fsmb.org.

Board certification in family medicine, internal medicine, or pediatrics are the most common certifications for primary care physicians. State boards also post public information about anything derogatory filed against physicians and board actions taken against physicians such as suspending or revoking their licenses.

When looking at the educational backgrounds of physicians you are considering, it is important to know that graduating from a prestigious medical school (such as Harvard) or a particular residency training program does not correlate with quality of medical care, health outcomes, or patient satisfaction. Also, the number of years of experience in medical practice is consistently associated favorably with patient satisfaction.

Given the fact that most physicians are medically qualified in their area of specialty, you will want to consider other factors in your selection process. How about reputation? Doctors' reputations reflected by online reviews and personal referrals are often useful in identifying potential primary care doctors. Google Reviews is actually a valid source to gauge satisfaction with a physician's service and quality of care. As you probably know from shopping for other products and services, you can expect a vocal (and angry) minority, but the weight of reviews should be glowing and submitted over a long period of time. Several other online review sites

(Healthgrades, RateMD, Vitals) take paid advertisements from doctors raising questions about objectivity.

Finally, people who are highly satisfied with their doctors tend to brag about them to their friends and family. If you ask your friends and family who they use as their primary care physicians, you will learn a lot. They will typically love their doctor—but hate their office. If you find friends who are highly impressed with the access to their doctor, the care and the efficiency of the office, that's one to consider. If you hear those compliments about a particular practice from multiple people, you're really onto something.

These personal referrals often provide much more detailed information about a physician than any published information can and therefore build more confidence in pursuing that physician or medical practice.

## Availability and Access

A brilliant, well-trained, experienced, friendly, licensed physician in good standing with the state who was referred to you by multiple friends and takes your insurance is completely worthless if they aren't available.

Arguably the most important and difficult quality to find in a primary care physician is that they be available to you when you need them. As I have detailed previously, America has a current and predicted future shortage of primary care physicians. We also have a majority of doctors whose schedules are overloaded and who are working in a system that has created great obstacles to timely care.

Is it possible to find a doctor who will talk with you on the phone today and can deliver same-day or next-day appointments whenever they are needed? Will visits with the doctor be rushed, or does the office schedule as much time as might be needed to address medical concerns? I assure you that, even though it is not the norm, it is possible and reasonable to expect time and attention.

When considering a new medical practice and doctor, you should press them to disclose their record on timely patient access and doctor availability. A potential primary care practice should be able to answer these questions to the satisfaction of anyone considering that practice:

- What is the current wait to schedule a routine preventive visit? How many days?
- Can an appointment with the preferred physician be scheduled today or tomorrow?
- How much time is allotted for an appointment?
- May I discuss several complaints with the doctor at the same visit?
- How long should I expect to wait in the waiting room(s) before I see the doctor?
- Can I talk with my doctor over the phone (during office hours and after hours)?
- Does the physician offer virtual visits via phone and video chat?
- Can I text and email my doctor directly?
- Do you provide patients with the doctor's personal cell phone number?

It is my belief that extreme availability and timely access are the most important prerequisites in choosing a primary care physician. If you can't reach your doctor right away to get answers now, nothing else matters. You should ask the practice manager or another administrative patient advocate your questions on this topic until you are comfortable that you know what you can expect in terms of access to the specific doctor you may choose.

Ideally, you will have high-level access to the one doctor who knows you best. If you can't be assured of this, you might decide to settle for reasonably timely access to someone/anyone else in the practice such as other physicians, nurse practitioners, or physician's assistants. Besides inquiring within the medical practice itself, try to discover answers about ease of access mentioned in online reviews and directly from friends and family who use that doctor or practice.

## Breadth of Services and Location

Timely access to your doctor is key. The convenience of a medical practice is also directly related to the accessibility of the doctor's office and the availability of various other medical services such as x-rays and labs that you may eventually need. When establishing a relationship with a new primary care physician, it is important to understand what types of medical services are available on-site in the doctor's office and what kinds of medical services you would have to be referred out for, if they are needed.

Most patients associate the convenience and value of a primary care practice not only with the office location's proximity to their home or work but also with common tests and treatments that are available in-house. Some independent medical practices are stripped down, offering little more than a place for a doctor to interview and examine patients. Others, typically practices that are owned by hospitals, are equipped with a broad array of additional services and specialists and may even be located in the hospital building or adjacent doctors' building.

While the breadth of additional services offered within your doctor's office may not be the driving factor in your selection, it is important to know how the practice deals with providing or referring for various services. Does the practice have in-office availability for blood drawing, laboratory blood tests, rapid strep (throat) tests, rapid influenza (flu) tests, COVID-19 (SARS-CoV-2) testing, a full array of CDC-recommended vaccines, vision and hearing screening, lung function testing, electrocardiogram (EKG), treadmill stress tests, x-rays, and surgical procedures (ability to suture or place stitches, wart/mole/cyst/skin tag removal, for example)?

Some primary care offices also offer on-site consultations with dietitians, diabetes educators, fitness trainers, and counselors/psychologists. For any of these services that are not provided within the doctor's office, it is important to understand how the practice deals with outside referrals.

Most people looking for a primary care physician also place the physical location of the office near the top of their selection criteria list. The location of the office should obviously be a consideration, but an inefficient practice that is always running late may negate the benefit of an office that is conveniently located. Driving five minutes to wait an hour for a five-minute visit with the doctor is likely more frustrating and inconvenient than driving twenty minutes for a five-minute wait and twenty or thirty minutes face-to-face with a doctor that you like. A few extra minutes of travel time may be well worth it if the practice across town runs more efficiently with minimal waiting. Or a suburban office might offer easy parking instead of a complicated parking ramp and long walks to reach medical offices in huge medical complexes.

## Personal Rapport

Do you like your doctor? For the vast majority of people, it is simply not enough that their doctor is knowledgeable and experienced at treating their medical conditions. It also doesn't matter if they are one of the rare doctors who can be highly accessible and available whenever you need them if you don't "like" them. A positive patient experience and high level of satisfaction has been shown to be more closely related to the relationship that someone has with their doctor than any other determinant.

*Do I like this doctor?* may be the most important question someone can ask when screening for a primary care physician. The bedside manner, personality, and communication skills of the doctor will reveal their level of interest in their patients and, therefore, the amount of effort they are likely to put forth in building a relationship of trust with you. This interest along with excellent communication skills and a propensity to educate their patients results in more time with each patient. More time leads to better understanding of their situations, more accurate diagnoses, better explanations, and greater clarity about recommendations.

Does the doctor seem to respect their patients and partner with them in decision-making or do they dictate action plans or belittle their patient's ideas and questions? How do you define a good working relationship with a doctor?

You wouldn't hire a handyman, a lawn service, or any other employee without an interview. You should not be expected to commit to a doctor-patient relationship with a primary care physician that you intend to stay with for a long time without first being given the opportunity to talk with them. Anyone looking for a new primary care physician should ask the medical practice for an opportunity to meet the physician to get to know them and their approach to patients before committing to ongoing care at that practice.

Forward-thinking medical practices will allow you some kind of no-obligation visit for this purpose. (But don't expect to receive medical advice or services without paying for them.) Most people are able to draw a conclusion quickly about the doctor's communication skills, demeanor, patience, and bedside manner, if simply given the opportunity to meet and interview the physician candidate.

Without this important step, many people end up wasting time jumping from doctor to doctor each time they have a medical need before landing with one that they actually like. Very inefficient. If you are in need of a new primary care physician, ask to meet the doctor for this purpose before being seen for any medical needs.

## Value

What is a good working relationship with a primary care physician worth? What is the value of having a doctor you like, who knows you, and is always available? The final important determining factor to consider here is the overall value of a stable primary care relationship.

Frankly, the only reason to go through the process outlined in this chapter for evaluating and selecting a doctor is to land with a physician who is more likely to deliver overall value to you over time. Will your new doctor provide services that are consistently important and useful to you, that you will appreciate and hold as having high intrinsic worth? People who are the most satisfied with their primary care doctors value the trust that they have in their advice (and availability) as well as the peace of mind the relationship gives them. This is the kind of value that the right primary care physician should provide.

Value also speaks to what you get for what it costs. When it comes to medical care, you pay in multiple ways. Even if your health insurance is provided by your employer at little or no direct price to you, it contains costs that you pay. Since your employer pays a significant portion if not all of your insurance premiums, they have less resources left to pay your salary or hourly wage. This benefit, in one way or another, decreases your take-home pay. You will also pay out of your pocket for deductibles, copayments (including primary care doctors' office visit copays), the cost of prescription and over-the-counter medications, and many other possibly excluded medical services. A primary care physician who recognizes and can have an influence on containing these kinds of additional expenses will deliver enhanced value directly to you.

Choosing a Direct Primary Care physician as your doctor is most likely to give you high overall value and satisfaction with care. Hundreds of thousands of patients from coast to coast have discovered the benefits and cost savings of a stable long-term relationship with a value-based DPC physician who is available when needed and has ample time to adequately address their needs. DPC practices are inherently more efficient and deliver quality care and cost savings simultaneously.

Health insurance does not guarantee access to healthcare, and the real cost of healthcare includes not only insurance premiums, office visit charges, copays, deductibles, lab costs, imaging costs, and more, but your time. You can't afford to waste time in unnecessary in-office visits, waiting for the doctor or seeking other clinics and hospitals when your primary physician is not available. These issues are largely eliminated with value-based Direct Primary Care arrangements.

## Find Your Next Doctor

I hope you have heard something new about what to look for when researching and selecting a primary care physician. Please use this chapter as a framework to identify the numerous important characteristics found in primary care physicians and practices that provide high levels of care, access, and value. If you are in the market for a doctor right now, you may want to get out pen and paper and list these characteristics or determining factors in order of greatest importance to you. Then start researching doctors in your area. Ask your friends and family for their experience and any suggestions they may have.

Then search online for "primary care physicians near me" or "direct primary care doctors" or "DPC doctors" in your town. If you believe that a value-based Direct Primary Care doctor may be right for you, a nationwide directory of more than 1,500 DPC practices is found at https://mapper.dpcfrontier.com/.

For each of your initial potential doctors, read their websites, online profiles, and patient/customer reviews. Which practices and doctors stand out? Do any of them emphasize the characteristics that you prioritized? Are any of those the same physicians that your friends or family endorsed? Now, start dialing.

If you can't get a human on the phone quickly or if no one calls you back, they are unlikely to be a practice that values communication and timely access. If you can get a manager or someone on the phone who can answer your questions favorably, then ask if they can provide a brief time for you to meet the doctor in person. When you get to that point, you are well on your way to making a well-informed choice in a new doctor!

In the next chapter I consider what to look for in a major medical insurance plan that will complement your choice of physician. Even if your insurance options are dictated by your employer and regardless of whether you choose a participating provider or an out-of-network DPC physician, it is important to understand the implications of various insurance plans on your costs and the efficiency of working with your new primary care doctor.

# 10

# Choosing Health Insurance to Complement DPC

Direct Primary Care guarantees you high-level access to the care you are most likely to use on a regular basis, but you still need health insurance.

If you choose to become a member of a Direct Primary Care practice, your DPC physician agrees to provide you with all or most primary care services for an affordable flat monthly fee. It is important to understand that (according to the majority of state laws) DPC payment arrangements are not health insurance. Patients who enter into services agreements with DPC physicians are purchasing access to a defined list of primary care services that all fall within the scope of practice normally delivered by family doctors. Because you don't want your family doctor to perform cardiac bypass surgery on you, replace your hip, or manage your cancer, you need a major medical health insurance plan of some kind to cover specialty care, hospitalizations, surgeries, and any other expensive and unpredictable health needs that might surprise you.

Your current health often dictates the most efficient approach to health insurance coverage. If you are generally healthy, you will not be admitted to a hospital, require a major surgery, or even need to see a specialist physician during most years. And if your doctor is a Direct Primary Care physician, your health insurance may go completely unused. You hope this is the case.

If you have been diagnosed with a serious medical condition and are being followed by one or more specialists, you probably already know and expect that you will be spending money out of your pocket for your care. Hopefully these medical care expenses are applied to your insurance deductible. You may even be likely to hit your deductible and maximum out-of-pocket payment responsibility more years than not. In these cases, richer insurance is desirable to offset high expected medical expenses. It is obviously important to consider your current health or preexisting conditions when deciding on a health insurance approach, but several other circumstances should also influence your decision.

In this chapter, I review general concepts of what types and amounts of coverage you should be looking for in an insurance plan to best complement the services that are provided by a DPC physician. I will also consider insurance options available to you when offered through an employer as well as other insurance plans that you can purchase directly as an individual or family.

Buying your own health insurance on the individual market most often occurs in situations where you are self-employed or when your employer does not offer an attractive insurance plan at a reasonable price or does not offer health benefits to employees at all. Of course, you may also be buying your own health insurance through government programs such as Medicare, Medicaid, or military insurance programs.

## Conceptually

I have demonstrated several advantages of using a DPC physician exclusively for all your primary care needs. Knowing that the medical services you are most likely to need in a given year are covered under the services agreement that you have with your DPC doctor will usually change what you are trying to accomplish with insurance and what you will be looking for in a plan.

Securing guaranteed, timely access to your doctor makes it much less likely that you will need to receive care from specialists, and, in most cases, the number and amounts of claims against your insurance policy will go down. Of course, your out-of-pocket costs for office visits, copayments, and deductibles will also go down. That means there is generally less risk that needs to be covered by an insurance plan for anyone who has entered into a services agreement with a DPC doctor, so choosing a less expensive insurance plan is frequently beneficial.

From a financial standpoint, the only thing worse than being underinsured is being overinsured. Conceptually, when choosing major medical insurance as a companion to a DPC arrangement, it is best to avoid paying for insurance coverage that duplicates reimbursement for services that you have already secured directly through your DPC doctor. Any time you have duplicate coverage through your insurance plan and also from your doctor, you are simply paying twice. To the degree that you can select a less expensive plan that makes primary care visits and services primarily the patient's responsibility, you will be making your overall coverage more efficient and saving yourself money in insurance premiums, deductibles, and copayments.

Since the advent of employer-sponsored major medical insurance benefits during and following World War II, the road to researching and selecting insurance is determined by whether or not someone is employed and if their employer offers health insurance. The Affordable Care Act requires that businesses with fifty or more full-time employees offer health insurance to their employees or pay a hefty penalty to the IRS. The plans offered must meet certain minimum requirements for coverage and affordability and must also be offered to dependents (children under the age of twenty-six) of employees.

Of course, there are many reasons that smaller businesses with fewer than fifty full-time employees also choose to offer health insurance. Health insurance benefits have been shown to be important to the vast majority of employees, create loyalty to the employer, improve stability and job longevity within the workforce, and may even be the sole reason that some employees stay in a job.

According to data from the Kaiser Family Foundation, about 50% of the entire US population participates in group insurance plans through their employer. Employers pay for the majority of the insurance cost leaving workers to pay an average of 17% of the premium for single coverage and 27% for family coverage. Logically, employees of companies offering health benefits should first consider whether these plans meet their needs before researching other alternatives.

For individuals who are not eligible for coverage through their employer or a spouse's employer, the hunt may require more effort, but a broader array of options and approaches is available. Sometimes, age or life circumstances make enrollment in a government-subsidized health insurance plan obvious. Medicare, Medicaid, and military health insurance covers 35% of all Americans, and subsidized ACA plans offered through health insurance marketplaces (exchanges) cover an additional 9.6 million people.

Let's consider what to look for in the many types of plans that may be offered through employers and those that are directly available to individuals and families on the private market.

## When Your Employer Offers Insurance

A full 50% of you reading this book currently have health insurance through your employer or the employer of a family member. There are several significant advantages of employer-sponsored health insurance. Employers typically pay the majority of the cost of insurance premiums while the employee on average pays less than one-fourth of the cost. The employer researches, chooses, and maintains the relationship with the insurance company and broker. Also, the premium contributions from your employer are not subject to federal taxes, and your contributions may often be made pretax, which lowers your taxable income.

The types of insurance, funding sources, plan structures, and coverages as well as the portion of the cost of insurance paid by the employer versus the employee all vary greatly. Let's briefly look at the breadth of group insurance types most commonly offered by employers and then consider how to make sense of and choose from the particular plans that your employer may offer if you choose to see a Direct Primary Care doctor.

- **Health Maintenance Organization (HMO)**: An HMO plan is generally one of the least expensive plan types with lower premiums and lower out-of-pocket costs. However, it also allows fewer choices in participating physicians and hospitals than other plans. Members are usually required to choose a participating primary care physician (PCP) to provide all of their initial care. A referral authorization from the PCP is required for the member to see any specialist physicians. In many cases, HMOs will cover a broader range of preventive services than other policies. Members are subject to copayments and may also have deductibles to meet before the plan will pay for certain services. Most HMO plans do not provide coverage for out-of-network providers without prior authorization from the PCP or in certain emergency situations.

- **Point of Service (POS)**: POS plans have some elements of HMO plans and some of PPO plans (discussed later). POS plans may require members to select a specific in-network PCP, and the care provided by the PCP isn't usually subject to a deductible. Specialty care is typically reimbursed at a higher rate if it can be provided by the PCP or if the PCP refers the member to a specialist. Services rendered by out-of-network providers are allowed but are subject to a deductible and lower level of coverage. In some cases, it is required that the member pay the entire bill at the time of service and then submit a claim for reimbursement. A POS plan provides somewhat more flexibility than an HMO plan but typically still requires a gatekeeper PCP for the member to receive the best coverage from specialists and out-of-network doctors and facilities.

- **Exclusive Provider Organization (EPO)**: EPO plans also require the selection of a primary care physician who will provide any needed referrals to in-network specialists. They are similar to HMO plans in that their members are required to use the plan's network of physicians, except in cases of emergency. EPO members are also responsible for modest copayments and may be subject to a deductible. EPOs usually have better choice in doctors (larger provider network) and hospitals than HMOs but do not have as large a physician network as PPOs. They are typically priced in between the cost of an HMO and a PPO.

- **Preferred Provider Organization (PPO)**: A PPO plan encourages members to use a network of preferred providers (doctors and hospitals) who have contracted with the insurance carrier to provide medical services to members of the plan at a discounted rate. Members may choose to see any doctors or specialists within the plan's network, and any services received outside of the network typically result in a higher out-of-pocket cost. PPO plans require that an annual deductible be met before the insurance company begins covering medical bills. Plans have individual and family deductibles as well as out-of-pocket maximum amounts that limit the amount that a member may have to pay for each contract year in various categories of coverage. Members are also responsible for fixed copayments for certain services such as office visits, ER visits, and imaging tests (x-ray, CT scan, MRI) or coinsurance payments of a fixed percentage of the total charges for other medical claims. Copays and coinsurance amounts are higher for services received from out-of-network providers.

- **High Deductible Health Plan (HDHP)**: An HDHP, by definition, has a higher deductible than other qualified insurance plans. HDHPs have lower monthly premiums but, since the deductible is higher, the member pays for more of the costs before insurance reimbursement kicks in. Members save money if they end up requiring less medical care but assume more of the financial risk on the front end. An HDHP can be an HMO, POS, PPO, or EPO. It may also be combined with Health Savings Accounts (HSA), Health Reimbursement Accounts (HRA), or Flexible Spending Accounts (FSA) that are discussed next. The IRS currently defines an HDHP as any plan with a deductible of at least $1,400 for an individual or $2,800 for a family. These plans also limit the maximum out-of-pocket expenses for in-network services to no more than $7,000 for an individual or $14,000 for a family.

- **HSAs, HRAs, and FSAs**: Health Savings Accounts, Health Reimbursement Accounts, and Flexible Spending Accounts are all types of accounts that may be offered by your employer in conjunction with any type of plan described above that is set up as a High Deductible Health Plan. These accounts vary in design, intended uses, how they are funded, and how they may be spent on healthcare services. An HSA is a bank account owned by an individual that may be used to pay for "qualified medical expenses." The owner/employee and/or the employer may put money into the HSA according to IRS guidelines. An HRA is an account that is owned and funded by the employer that reimburses employees for qualified medical expenses. These reimbursements to employees are usually tax-free. FSAs are also accounts held by the employer for their employees to pay for many out-of-pocket medical expenses with tax-free dollars. FSAs are funded by the employee at an amount that they choose in pretax dollars, up to a limit set by the employer. Any money not spent on healthcare expenses by the end of the year may be spent in the first 2.5 months of the following year or a maximum of $500 may be carried into the next year. Otherwise, unused funds are forfeited.

Whew! If all of these acronyms seem overwhelming and difficult to tell apart, you're not alone. To make matters even more confusing, there are numerous other types of insurance and health benefits that employers may offer—but I won't cover them here. The preceding section covers all of the most common types of employer-sponsored insurance.

Fortunately, if you are considering health insurance offered through your employer, you only need to fully understand the terms of the specific options that your employer chooses. And if your employer is like most, they will offer more than one option and will be paying the majority of the cost for your insurance policy. That means it should be clear as you look at the amount you will pay (your contribution) that at least one of the plans your employer offers is likely to provide clear value to you. You probably take it.

Let's consider what's important when choosing a plan to best complement an arrangement with a Direct Primary

Care physician. Two general categories will determine your priorities in selecting a company-sponsored insurance plan. Either you are generally healthy and never go to the doctor (or infrequently enough that you use that phrase), or you have been diagnosed with one or more significant medical conditions that require you to be treated on a regular basis by one or more physician specialists. The category that you fall into should direct your selection of insurance.

If you have historically gone to the doctor infrequently and your medical costs have been low, you are likely to save money over the years by choosing the least expensive insurance option offered to you. Ideally, it will be some sort of High Deductible Health Plan that is light on first-dollar coverages and mostly focused on providing catastrophic coverage. You are likely to be able to save more money on your contribution to this type of insurance plan's premiums than you will spend on your primary care in a given year.

If you have a DPC physician, you don't need coverage for primary care office visits and are likely to be able to pay the DPC doctor's membership fees, heavily discounted prices for lab tests, imaging (x-ray, CT scans, MRI), and generic prescription medications and still save money over the cost of a "Cadillac" insurance plan.

If it is presented as an option, you should also seriously consider the value of adding an HSA, HRA, or FSA. Each of these accounts has its own characteristics, but are all designed to be used to pay for (or to reimburse you for) certain healthcare expenses for you and your covered dependents. In some cases, these funds may be used to pay for DPC membership fees and other services provided by your DPC physician. The IRS rules for accessing these accounts for DPC services are evolving and somewhat confusing.

The US House of Representatives and US Senate have taken up legislation that would clarify the IRS code to define DPC arrangements as qualified medical expenses and officially endorse their use in conjunction with HDHPs and HSAs. When considering using any of these accounts to pay for DPC fees, it is best to review your intended use with your company's benefits director and your personal tax adviser.

If, on the other hand, you are being followed frequently by medical specialists for one or more significant medical conditions and can predict that your medical expenses will be high year in and year out, you may benefit from more insurance. A plan that is more expensive but offers a lower deductible and better coverages for the kinds of care you know you will need may actually save you money over a cheaper plan and will certainly provide peace of mind, making it more likely to predict how much your care will cost you directly in a given year.

High Deductible Health Plans may also be reasonable options with the knowledge that you may be paying for all of your medical costs until the deductible is met. Once the out-of-pocket maximum expense under the plan has been met, all covered expenses should be paid for by the plan. As long as this is clearly understood and is acceptable within your budget, these plans may be worth considering.

Maintaining a relationship with a Direct Primary Care physician will represent a small fraction of your overall healthcare and health insurance expense and contributes great value in terms of fast access, meeting your primary care needs, coordinating the care or your specialists, and in being available to help explain your medical conditions and treatments when specialists aren't available or don't have the time.

## When You Are Buying Your Own

Just over 41% of Americans have health insurance that they purchase as individuals or as families and not as part of an employer's group insurance plan. The greatest number of these people are enrolled in government-run insurance: Medicare (14.2% of the total population), Medicaid (19.8%), and military (1.4%). Only 5.9% of people in the country are covered by privately purchased nongovernment-run nongroup health insurance, and about two-thirds of these have purchased a plan through the federal health insurance marketplace. An explanation of federal and state health insurance programs is beyond the scope of this book. It is my experience that many people who have Medicare, Medicaid, and military insurance coverage find it difficult to get care when they need it and find that maintaining a relationship with a Direct Primary Care doctor to be well worth the small additional cost.

Let's look at marketplace ACA Obamacare plans, individual insurance that may be purchased outside of the health insurance marketplace, and alternatives to traditional health insurance coverage such as medical cost-sharing arrangements.

The federal health insurance marketplace or exchange is an online shopping website (healthcare.gov) where numerous healthcare plans are offered to individuals. These plans are sold by private health insurance carriers and meet the requirements of the Affordable Care Act (ACA, also called Obamacare), covering all essential health benefits including hospital care, outpatient services, emergency services, maternity care, mental health, substance abuse treatment, prescription drug coverage, lab services, and rehabilitative services. The website allows individuals to browse and compare these qualified health plans and to purchase them during certain open enrollment windows each year.

Qualifying plans are also available through private online marketplaces as well as insurance marketplaces currently offered by twenty-one states. The ACA also created premium tax credits, which are subsidies issued by the federal government to offset the cost of insurance premiums for policies purchased through the marketplace/exchange to individuals who qualify based on need and estimated annual income. People who are offered health insurance through their employer generally do not qualify for any subsidies.

Prior to COVID-19, that vast majority (84%) of individuals enrolled in ACA plans were already receiving these tax credits. A new COVID-19 relief law, the American Rescue Plan Act of 2021, has significantly increased the percentage of applicants who qualify for premium tax credits as well as the amount of premium reductions that they receive. Suffice it to say that if you are one of the many unemployed or self-employed individuals who qualify for these reduced-cost insurance plans, it is likely to be your most affordable option for comprehensive insurance coverage. The amount of your premium reduction will also more than likely exceed the cost of a membership with a DPC physician. This pairing of a qualified ACA-subsidized plan along with a DPC arrangement should assure you of high-level access to your personal primary care doctor along with reasonable insurance coverage for any unexpected or expensive medical needs.

Another option for individuals who find the marketplace plans too costly, who do not qualify for significant premium tax credits, or who don't feel it is necessary to carry a traditional comprehensive insurance policy are individual health insurance plans of many types and plan designs that may be purchased outside of the exchanges.

As of 2019, the ACA individual mandate that previously required all Americans to carry health insurance that met the law's definition of essential health benefits was effectively repealed by Congress. Americans are now free to purchase whatever degree and type of insurance that is available on the private market without any tax penalty, unless it is required by their state of residence. Currently, only California, Rhode Island, Massachusetts, New Jersey, and the District of Columbia have requirements for minimum essential coverage and penalties if you don't have it.

Among nonqualified health insurance plans are fixed-indemnity plans, short-term health insurance, limited benefit plans, Farm Bureau plans, travel insurance, and accident supplements. These types of plans are generally cheaper on the front end but don't have broad comprehensive coverage and may leave you on the hook for substantial medical expenses.

If you determine that you should consider alternatives to ACA qualified health plans, it is recommended that you consult with an independent health insurance agent/broker who can advise you about your options. An agent/broker can also present choices of High Deductible Health Plans that may or may not be considered ACA-compliant plans but may be designed in such a way as to optimally complement Direct Primary Care services.

Another alternative to traditional insurance plans that has been expanding rapidly in the US since 2010 is medical cost-sharing plans. These plans are not insurance and are not regulated as insurance in most states. A medical cost-sharing plan is a low-cost alternative to traditional health insurance that functions as a cooperative in which members contractually agree to "share" certain (more expensive) medical bills. These plans are promoted under various names such as medical cost sharing, healthcare cost sharing, healthshare plans, healthcare sharing ministries, Christian health share, and more.

They are often made up of members who are like-minded in some way, and many are faith-based. Most will require members to agree to certain standards or core values and to agree to live a healthy lifestyle in order to participate.

The Alliance of Health Care Sharing Ministries states that the US Department of Health and Human Services has certified 108 such organizations that collectively have 1.5 million participants in all fifty states and share $1.3 billion in medical expenses each year. Limitations of these plans include that they do not guarantee reimbursement for medical expenses, generally do not cover preexisting conditions (during the first year of participation) or preventive care, are not regulated as insurance, and hold few legal protections for members. However, they have generally proven to be reliable and are attractive due to high reimbursement or sharing limits and their significantly lower cost than traditional insurance plans.

Medical cost-sharing plans have become popular with people who are committed to receiving their primary care through a Direct Primary Care (DPC) physician and want to add inexpensive protection that covers high-dollar catastrophic healthcare costs. In fact, many of these plans recognize the value of DPC in terms of reduction of downstream healthcare costs and provide credits or discounts on their fees for participants who are also patients of DPC practices. Examples of some of the more prominent plans include Christian Healthcare Ministries, Medi-Share, Samaritan Ministries, Liberty HealthShare, Zion Health, Sedera Healthshare, One Share Health, Altrua Healthshare, Solidarity Healthshare, and

Trinity Healthshare. These plans are sold directly online and also through certain health insurance agents/brokers.

## From My Practice

You may recall my patient Matt (from chapter 3). Matt is a sixty-one-year-old patient of mine who had too many doctors, too many specialists, and too much money going to health insurance premiums. When he joined my DPC practice, he was able to prune back many of his physician specialists, but he was still paying a lot of money for a health insurance policy that would cover all of his high medical bills. Since he now had an accessible primary care physician to manage his current risks and medical conditions, he no longer needed most of his specialty physicians. He felt he now had too much insurance.

Matt is self-employed, made just over $100,000 last year, and was paying about $1,100 per month for an ACA marketplace silver plan. He had a zero-dollar deductible but wasn't receiving any tax credits (discounts) due to his high income. When he was seeing several specialist physicians, he was glad that he didn't have a deductible, but since getting rid of those other doctors, he anticipated having very little out-of-pocket medical expenses most years and wanted to look for a cheaper insurance plan, even if it meant having a deductible.

In 2021, the American Rescue Plan Act changed the premium tax credit calculations to grant subsidies to people with higher incomes. With this change, Matt was able to get an ACA bronze EPO plan with a $6,000 deductible for $559 per month—about half of what he had been paying. With the premium tax credit discount, even after he pays me for his primary care services ($105 per month), he saves about $5,000 per year compared with what he paid for the insurance plan alone the previous year. Unless he hits his full $6,000 deductible four out of five years, he is saving money and simultaneously securing unrestricted access to his personal primary care doctor.

## Pick Insurance that Pairs with DPC

Any way you slice it, choosing health insurance for you and your family is generally complicated and usually feels overwhelming. It is invariably more expensive than you think it should be and leaves you sharing some version of risk. You will either choose an expensive high-end plan that covers nearly all your medical expenses but wonder if you wasted money on more extensive coverage than you needed, or you will try to save money on some sort of limited and inexpensive plan that causes you to be exposed to more financial risk and expense if you are surprised by surgery, hospitalization, or a serious medical diagnosis.

If you plan to lock into an affordable membership with a DPC physician to guarantee coverage of your primary care needs, it can simplify and narrow your major medical insurance choices. If you are healthy, you will want to look for less expensive policies with higher deductibles, betting that you won't have significant unexpected medical expenses most years. In these cases, a more affordable high-deductible plan will often save you more than you pay for your DPC membership.

If you have significant medical conditions or substantial anticipated medical bills each year, you may choose a richer plan with lower deductibles and copayments. Even in these cases, a relationship with a DPC doctor who knows you and is always available will deliver significant value for all of the reasons previously discussed.

Finally, you should ask a lot of questions. If insurance is being offered through your employer, ask your human resources manager or company health benefits agent to explain the details, pros and cons, of every option they are making available. If you are searching for insurance as an individual or family, an independent health insurance adviser, agent, or broker can be a valuable source for answers during your process. Fortunately, these choices are never fatal or final. You are most often committing for one year and are free to readjust your plan and approach next year, if needed.

# PART IV

# EMPLOYEE HEALTH FROM THE CARE UP

# 11

# Direct Primary Care for Employers and Employees

Let's look at healthcare and health insurance from the employer's perspective.

In this chapter and the next, I consider employee health benefits, actual employee health, and the financial ramifications of both from the perspective of the employer. If you are a business owner, executive, middle manager, human resources specialist, or otherwise have budgetary responsibility at your company, the following insights should be helpful to your understanding of this important aspect of your business.

At the end of the day, every business is a healthcare business. Health benefits are typically the second or third largest line item in a company's budget, so *your* healthcare business is indeed big business.

Businesses spend so much on health insurance for several reasons. Primarily, because it's expected. The employer mandate contained within the Affordable Care Act requires all businesses with fifty or more full-time employees to provide affordable insurance that meets minimum requirements or face hefty penalties. Health insurance coverage is also expected by employees, regardless of whether or not their employer is legally required to provide it. This employee benefit is nearly essential in order to attract and retain high-quality employees for the long run. The quality of health coverage and the direct cost to employees matter to them. A generous benefits package that offers health insurance with good coverage and doesn't cost employees too much out of their paychecks or pocket is attractive during recruiting and has been shown to be a significant factor in employee longevity with their employer.

The COVID-19 pandemic also created new pressures on employers. In addition to shaky revenue and new expenses, there have been new operational challenges, a shift to remote work, and a pivot of business offerings to preserve viability. Initially, employees were worried about keeping their jobs. Now, employers are worried about finding employees who want to work for an acceptable rate of pay. These changes in the available workforce have employers rethinking compensation packages, including health benefits, as a means to attract and keep quality employees in a post-pandemic environment.

Group health insurance is expensive and getting more expensive. I have discussed the current drivers of skyrocketing health insurance prices and what can be done to curtail them. As you might imagine by now, Direct Primary Care can play a significant role in reducing healthcare costs and thereby suppressing health insurance costs while simultaneously creating value and loyalty in employees.

In this chapter I propose a paradigm shift in how employers look at providing health benefits. This new paradigm is for companies to build their health benefits from the care up. Rather than simply providing a group insurance plan that does not assure access to care, they should consider guaranteeing their employees unrestricted access to primary care services through Direct Primary Care doctors as the foundation of their health benefits package. With this most frequently needed care in place, employers may then build upon the DPC foundation by selecting or designing a group insurance plan that most closely complements the services already covered most affordably by DPC physicians.

## Why Does Your Company Offer Health Benefits?

In other words, what's in it for your company? What is your business hoping to accomplish by providing health benefits to its employees? If you haven't thought about it and don't have a strategic plan for your healthcare business, you are potentially wasting a lot of money on that huge line item in your budget. Health benefits offerings should benefit both the employer and the employees. There should be an explicit and measurable return on investment (ROI) for the business and also significant perceived and actual value received by the workforce members who participate. Let's consider what's in it for employers and employees.

Why do employers offer health insurance and other health benefits? Couldn't they simply pay employees more in hourly rate or salary and let them buy their own individual or family medical insurance? We know that employers with more than fifty full-time employees are obligated by law to provide this benefit, but there are multiple compelling reasons to do so, even when it isn't required. These factors directly and indirectly benefit the employer and their bottom line. When done right, providing quality health benefits is a substantial and important investment in the business. Optimizing health benefits for employees can result in all of the following measurable outcomes that accrue to the health and profitability of the business as well as the health and happiness of employees.

- **Lower Insurance Premiums**: Throughout the history of group insurance plans, they have generally been less expensive than the individual plans that employees could purchase on their own. Purchasing discounted insurance may provide value to the employer, which can be used as a type of currency to compensate and invest in employees.

- **Insurance Premiums Are Tax Deductible**: Businesses can deduct 100% of the cost of health insurance premiums from federal corporate taxes. Some small businesses with fewer than twenty-five employees may also qualify for a Small Business Health Care Tax Credit, which is worth as much as 50% of the costs a small business pays for their employees' health insurance premiums.

- **Valuable Recruiting Tool**: The perk of good health insurance options as part of a generous benefits package is appealing to potential new employees. They greatly value employee benefits in addition to their salary or hourly pay rate. Health insurance is of particular value to employees because a significant portion of the insurance premiums is typically paid by the employer, and the employee's contribution (if any) is often paid before taxes are withheld. When individuals purchase health insurance on their own, they pay in after-tax dollars and, of course, are responsible for 100% of a larger premium.

- **Employee Loyalty and Retention**: Healthcare benefits remain important to employees over time. Offering attractive medical benefits increases loyalty in valued employees and has been shown to improve employee retention and longevity. A 2019 survey by Transamerica Center for Health Studies revealed that 51% of employed adults indicated that they have to stay at their current job for the health insurance and 30% said they had previously left a job because their company did not offer adequate health benefits. High-value health benefits improve employee retention, which directly benefits the corporate bottom line by reducing the substantial switching costs of recruiting, hiring, and training new employees.

- **Job Satisfaction**: Health insurance is one important component of overall employee job satisfaction. According to surveys by Employee Benefit Research Institute, 80% of employees who say they have good healthcare benefits have high job satisfaction while only 25% of employees who are dissatisfied with health benefits report that they are loyal to their employer.

- **Employee Health**: Healthy employees are more productive and more likely to be happy. They exhibit less absenteeism, take fewer sick days, are better able to focus on tasks, and retain important information.

> Reliable and timely access to a primary care physician (even a telehealth visit during the workday where the employee doesn't have to leave the job) also improves health and minimizes days and hours away from work.

Good health benefits, including easy access to a personal primary care physician, have been proven to deliver all of the benefits just listed to employers and employees. Not only do these factors improve morale and productivity, they also make it possible for companies to spend less on healthcare and more on growing their business. Specifically, investing in access to primary care for employees has been shown to have a beneficial effect on total healthcare and health insurance costs for employers (as explained in chapter 8). More primary care equals less expense.

What's in it for your employees? What do employees value the most in health benefits? Ultimately, they want what you want—value. They want the greatest amount of protection and coverage for their expected and potentially unpredictable medical care for the least cost. They want excellent access to the care they need, when they need it, for as little as possible in out-of-pocket costs. They want low insurance premiums, low deductibles, and low copayments for all services. When asked, they are consistently most focused on common day-to-day medical expenses—the things they are most likely to need most often. They want to pay as little as possible for primary care office visits, lab tests, prescription medications, for example, and to be able to get them with as little effort as possible.

What do patients value most in their doctor? There have been many patient surveys and published lists of patient expectations and the qualities they are looking for in a doctor. The boildown is that patients are looking for these four qualities they value the most:

1. **Time**: Patients want to spend more time with their doctor. They want the doctor to listen. They want their doctor, in the words of Stephen Covey, to seek first to understand, then to be understood. They also simply want their doctor to be available. They want an appointment today. They want to be able to talk to the doctor on the phone—today. Especially in post-pandemic America, they want to be able to text, email, and video chat with their doctor—today. Among the most frequent complaints people have about their doctor is that they are "always in a hurry" and "I can never get in to see them." It's all about T-I-M-E and timely access.

2. **An Advocate**: Patients highly value a navigator. The American healthcare system is complex and confusing. Patients typically recognize their need for a trusted adviser to guide them, to provide answers now for their health needs, and to direct them to the most necessary, efficient, and cost-effective care. Implicit in their desire for a doctor who is their advocate is the patient's need to be confident in their physician's objectivity and motives. It is crucial for patients to have a doctor whose incentives are fully aligned with the patient. They want a physician who doesn't benefit or profit based on the advice they give or the tests and treatments they prescribe.

3. **Communication**: Patients need to understand. In addition to valuing a doctor who listens, they are

looking for a personal physician who is a good communicator. Medical concepts and terminology are foreign to most people. Physicians who can explain the answers to the patient's questions, *What's wrong with me?* and *What should I do about it?* in a clear and effective manner, in everyday language, are not easy to come by and are more likely to deliver quality care with high patient satisfaction.

4. **Care**: Patients would actually like some care along with their healthcare. They want a doctor who is considerate and empathetic with a caring bedside manner. It is important to them that their doctor cares about them, seeks to get to know them, makes eye contact, and respects their opinions and decisions. They need a caring partner with whom to make shared decisions. As Teddy Roosevelt said, "Nobody cares how much you know until they know how much you care."

Is there a way to accomplish the goals of the employer and the employees at the same time? Can employer health benefits become a win-win that helps accomplish the triple aim of better care for employees, better health for the employer's workforce, and lower overall healthcare and health insurance costs for the employer and employees? Of course, you're reading a book that asserts that it's possible. But in order to get to a solution for ever-escalating healthcare and health insurance costs, we first need to understand why these costs are going up.

## Why Are Healthcare Costs Skyrocketing?

Employers and employees alike are now conditioned to expect health insurance and healthcare expenses in general to be very expensive and to rise every year, sometimes by double-digit percentages. According to Dave Chase in his book *Restoring the American Dream*, healthcare costs per se aren't actually rising. He asserts that the true costs of medical services (in a retail world without the complications of health insurance) are stable, and it is more correctly the prices of health insurance that are rising substantially, unnecessarily, and often nefariously.

While America's health insurance environment and the ways that we pay for healthcare are primary drivers of escalating healthcare costs, there are other important (and related) factors. One additional factor, which was covered in some detail in chapter 4 as it relates to a shortage of primary care physicians, is our country's aging population and their increased need for care. People over the age of sixty-five spend, on average, three times more per capita on healthcare services than younger adults and five times more than children. Containing costs in this population is obviously important, but the phenomenon is more of a reason than an excuse for increased costs.

Let's talk about the four major areas driving healthcare costs in which we should be able to effect positive change: technology is expensive, our health insurance system is broken, individual behavior and choices make people sicker, and there are significant issues with the delivery of primary care.

## *Technology Is Expensive*

Technology is expensive. Some estimates indicate that new medical technology and expanded adoption of medical technology contributes 40 to 50% to all healthcare cost increases we are experiencing today. Technological innovation has unquestionably improved our health and the treatment of illness, injury, and disease. Numerous innovations over the past several decades have produced vaccines, antibiotics, invasive cardiac care, advanced surgeries, and cancer treatments, as well as revolutionary health information technology.

A hundred years ago, your heart attack would be treated with the advice to "take two aspirin and call me in the morning." We all benefit from the fact that this is no longer the standard of care! Americans, particularly, place great value and hope in modern medicine and the technological advancements that continue to be introduced. Technology is an understandable and legitimate cause of increasing actual costs, and we would be ill advised to deter innovation in attempts to contain cost.

The goal should be to use technology to benefit the health of the greatest number of people while containing costs by utilizing the most advanced and expensive products and procedures efficiently and judiciously. Just because we can do a fancy test, perform a cutting-edge surgical technique, or prescribe the latest and greatest branded pharmaceuticals doesn't mean we should. Healthcare costs can appropriately be restrained by employing expensive technology appropriately in situations with clear and proven outcomes-based advantages when reasonable cost-benefit analyses are compelling.

## *Our Health Insurance System Is Broken*

Our health insurance system is broken. America doesn't have a healthcare crisis. We have a health insurance crisis and a reimbursement structure crisis and a cost-shifting crisis and a pricing deception crisis. Other than that, we're good.

The insurance-driven volume-based fee-for-service payment system that inserts multiple nonvalue-added middlemen between patients and providers has been well-documented to add substantial cost. In addition to inflating costs dramatically, the system creates significant misaligned incentives that are detrimental to the quality of patient care. A complete discussion of the problems with the American healthcare system is beyond the scope of this book (or any single book), but here is a brief list of the greatest issues:

- **Fee-for-service reimbursement** pays doctors more to bill more services, which incentivizes inappropriate overutilization of tests and treatments that drive up costs to employers and employees.

- **Cost-shifting policies** charge various patients different amounts for the same service, which causes some patients to pay above-market rates for services to offset losses that the provider sustains due to other contractual agreements.

- **Lack of price transparency** means that providers have not typically offered information in advance on the prices of services that they render so that services have often already been received and patients are later surprised by the cost only after the bill or Explanation of Benefits (EOB) arrives in the mail. To date, competitive pricing information is almost never available from multiple provider options so that the patient and employer would be able to compare and choose providers that offer the best prices and greatest value. Even with the Consolidated Appropriations Act (CAA) and "no surprise billing" set to go into effect in 2022, it remains to be seen if required pricing information disclosures will have a significant real-world effect on consumer choices and costs. There is also a detrimental and costly lack of transparency in the compensation of health insurance brokers. Employers are rarely aware of the degree to which the broker benefits from selling them a more costly insurance plan. Lack of transparency eliminates competition and consumer choice.

- **Drug pricing practices** are also a significant cause of escalating overall healthcare costs. Prescription medications comprise 10% of total healthcare spending in the US and are rising by 4 to 6% per year. The market for prescription drugs is very complex, also lacks transparency, and is riddled with anticompetitive business practices. These issues result in prices paid for brand-name medications and generics that are far higher than is necessary. There is also an excessively high amount of cost shifting in this area of the healthcare industry nationally.

- **Misaligned incentives** may cause employers to be presented with group insurance options that serve the interests of the carrier or insurance broker over those of the employer and employees. Who pays your broker? While many insurance agents/brokers present themselves as buyer's agents, they are paid by the insurance carriers and may act more like agents of the insurance companies. Their total compensation from the sale of insurance plans is often not disclosed to the customer, and they are paid more when the employer purchases richer plans. Another area of misaligned incentives is that when more claims are filed against the policy, premiums will be higher upon plan renewal, which further increases the carrier's profit as well as the broker's potential compensation. At a minimum, these incentives serve to maintain the status quo and make it less likely that brokers will be discussing innovative and beneficial changes that include Direct Primary Care.

- **Fraud and abuse in healthcare** is widespread and staggering. The FBI estimates losses due to healthcare fraud to be as high as $226 billion annually or 10% of total healthcare expenditures. Healthcare fraud is a felony and may be perpetrated by insurance plan members or by providers. Unfortunately, insurance carriers and their claims administrators are not highly motivated to catch fraudulent activity as more fraudulent claims drive up healthcare spending, which in turn results in increased premiums and insurance carrier profit.

- **Bloated administrative costs** add an enormous load to our healthcare system in America. A review of spending by insurers and providers in the US in 2017 revealed that 34.2% of total national health expenditures were spent on administrative costs. This equates to $812 billion or $2,497 for every person in America. The negative effects caused by our inefficient and complex third-party payer system with its numerous middlemen between doctors and patients cannot be overstated.

## *Individual Behavior Directly Increases Healthcare Costs*

What is the number one killer in America today? It's not heart disease, cancer, accidents, or COVID-19. The number one killer is procrastination. Putting off important preventive screenings for life-threatening conditions and not making healthy lifestyle choices are the root causes of countless diseases and premature deaths. The delayed detection and treatment of preventable conditions results in the need for significantly more healthcare services and expense. In this way, your employees' behaviors escalate their own healthcare costs and the company's.

Unhealthy lifestyle choices kill. Alcoholics die from alcohol. Smokers die from smoking. A significant number of the rest of us ultimately die from something related to what we eat, how much we weigh, and how much exercise we get. These lifestyle factors are major risk factors for cardiovascular disease (heart attack and stroke) and numerous types of cancer, which kill more Americans than all other causes combined.

The leading causes of preventable death are smoking, weight-related causes, and alcoholism. The CDC estimates that as many as 40% of deaths from major causes are premature, due to modifiable risk factors, and are, therefore, preventable. The cost of these lifestyle-related preventable diseases is shockingly high and is estimated at more than $730 billion per year in the US alone.

Disease is expensive. Advanced disease is worse. We know that preventive screening and early detection save lives. There is also good evidence that many preventive screening procedures save significant amounts of money. It is estimated that cost savings from early diagnosis of all cancers could be as much as $26 billion per year or 17% of total expenditures. Unfortunately, people are procrastinating or ignoring preventive screening recommendations. National results from the Preventive Services Self-Administered Questionnaire published in 2018 show that only 8.3% of adults over the age of thirty-five had received all high-priority preventive services, and about 5% had not received any of these services whatsoever.

A final area of individual behavior that significantly affects healthcare costs to employers and employees is a lack of knowledge about how to best access cost-effective and appropriate medical care. Without guidance from a health professional, people often inappropriately and unnecessarily overutilize urgent care clinics, hospital emergency departments, and specialist physicians. According to research published in 2019 by UnitedHealth Group, a full two-thirds of all ER visits are avoidable and not actual emergencies. This equates to 18 million visits per year and $32 billion in unnecessary cost for conditions that could have been managed in primary care offices.

People also regularly overspend on prescription medications without realizing that their medications (or equivalents) may be readily available for a small fraction of the cost they are paying through their pharmacy insurance benefits. A study from the University of Southern California concluded that the "copay clawback phenomenon," whereby commercially insured patients' copayments exceed the total cost that their insurer or pharmacy benefit manager pays for a drug, results in overpayment by patients in 23% of all prescriptions filled nationally.

Further, in the common case where individuals are paying for prescription drugs without insurance coverage, they also often overpay substantially due to lack of knowledge of readily available online medication discount services.

## *Inadequate Delivery of Primary Care*

Inadequate delivery of primary care services is a root cause of America's expensive and inefficient healthcare system. As detailed in Part II of this book, the current shortcomings of access to timely primary care frustrate patients/employees and contribute to the majority of other causes of increasing healthcare costs.

In the absence of effective primary care, people overutilize expensive high-tech solutions and specialty care, suffer from all of the inefficiencies and issues that are ubiquitous within our third-party reimbursement systems, do not receive effective ongoing disease management, and are less likely to address the drivers of disease by seeking preventive screenings and making needed healthy lifestyle changes.

Placing primary care under the umbrella of health insurance significantly increases primary care cost and cripples access. It simultaneously pushes additional unnecessary care and expense downstream to specialists whose care and interventions are much more costly.

Every one of these causes of skyrocketing healthcare costs needs to be addressed. Some of the largest dollar opportunities may be found in systemic reforms of specialty care and end-of-life care, but there is only one reform that is likely to have an impact on all four of the aforementioned drivers of inflated costs. It is fixing primary care. The most efficient and effective model to do this is Direct Primary Care. The volume-based primary care "canary" is dead in the insurance-mediated "coal mine."

In the next section, I introduce a paradigm that many believe is the first and foundational answer to overall healthcare reform and achievement of the triple aim.

## DPC as the Foundation of Health Benefits

Health insurance does not equal health care. If your company is like most, your decision-makers assume that the group health insurance policy is the foundation of all health benefits. An insurance plan may be your only health benefit. It has always been that way, and your broker or benefits consultant assures you that this is the only perspective that makes sense. You offer health insurance but leave the search for actual medical care to the motivation and luck of your employees.

If this is your approach, you've got it exactly upside down. Providing health insurance does not ensure that your employees will receive quality healthcare. Health insurance is designed and useful for expensive and unpredictable medical costs. However, the majority of your employees are generally healthy. For them, expensive and unpredictable medical care happens only rarely.

Primary care, on the other hand, is invariably inexpensive, predictable, and needed by every employee every year. In fact, about 90% of medical needs experienced by employees in a typical year are best handled by a primary care physician. The foundation of healthcare is primary care, but adequate and timely access to it isn't easy to find. Your benefits structure will function best when it aligns with each of these facts.

The best way to accomplish your goals for health benefits and those of your employees is to build your health benefits from the care up. Build on the foundation of guaranteeing your employees high-level access to their personal primary care physician whenever they need them. The foundation of health is proactive, preventive, and related to lifestyle choices and the consistent management of common conditions (such as blood pressure, cholesterol, and diabetes). It requires timely care and the avoidance of expensive and unnecessary specialty care.

Efficient use of the entire healthcare system by your employees also requires a trusted health adviser to direct them and help them navigate their care. Optimal and easy access to quality primary care is all of those things. When Direct Primary Care forms the foundation of your company's benefits package, your approach to paying for the major medical expenses and insurance of your employees can be adjusted and modified as circumstances require without disrupting the continuity of care that your employees have with their DPC physician. You can confidently tell your workforce that they can "keep their doctor."

DPC accomplishes every one of the goals that your company has for providing health benefits and delivers on each of the qualities that employees value most in health benefits and in their doctor. Employees perceive the aspects of enhanced care and access to their personal physician that they receive with DPC as premium benefits. Specifically, they greatly value time with their doctor, a high level of communication, advice in navigating the healthcare system, considerate care and unrestricted 24/7 access with no additional out-of-pocket expenses.

A DPC benefit to employees becomes a valuable recruiting tool, improves employee loyalty and retention, and has the potential to enhance job satisfaction and increase productivity. Of course, as shown previously, enhanced access to primary care services also unquestionably improves employee health.

Numerous benefits of DPC may alter and reduce your company's cost for major medical expenses and insurance. DPC changes the utilization of healthcare services. It increases primary care interactions but decreases overall insurance claims. By definition, no insurance claims are ever filed for DPC services. As mentioned, research has shown a significant decrease in claims for multiple specialty categories due to 24/7 access to primary care, a focus on preventive care, and more consistent disease management.

DPC reduces healthcare costs and, therefore, reduces the need for as high a level of insurance. Inasmuch as your employees' relationships with their DPC physicians change their behavior for the better in terms of lifestyle, preventive screening and appropriate utilization of the healthcare system in general, overall healthcare costs to your employees and your company will decrease. This effect creates a financial opportunity for the company to consider alternative sources of funding, including self-insurance.

## Care First, Then Insurance

Direct Primary Care is beneficial for employers and employees. It can form a logical and highly affordable foundation of a health benefits plan that will accomplish the objectives of your company and the needs of your employees. DPC is uniquely positioned to address each of the major drivers of escalating healthcare costs. Major medical costs that are expensive and unpredictable still need to be administrated and insured.

In the final chapter, I explore ways to approach paying for major medical expenses in light of the economies that DPC provides. Within our new paradigm, well-informed choices can reduce overall healthcare costs and contribute to your company's bottom line. I cover the selection of health insurance, how to approach self-funding, and discuss what to look for in an enlightened benefits consultant to help you through your strategic process.

# 12

# Employer Selection of Medical Insurance to Complement DPC

Should you select your health insurance plan or design it? In this final chapter, I look at the status quo for employer-sponsored group health insurance and consider a better way.

The five largest national health insurance carriers own and drive the majority of corporate health insurance business. The BUCAH carriers (Blue Cross, United, Cigna, Aetna, and Humana) have 169 million members across the US representing over 51% of the total population. In addition to fully insured group plans, they control nearly 70% of all employer self-funded plans. And 47% of covered workers in 2020 were participating in PPO plans, the most common plan type, and 31% currently have High Deductible Health Plans with a savings option (HDHP/SO). Another 13% have an HMO, 8% a POS plan, and 1% are enrolled in a conventional indemnity plan.

These insurance carriers market plans that are predefined, inflexible, and are often less than ideal for individual businesses. Fortunately for companies of all sizes, there are better options than simply picking from a list of canned BUCAH insurance options.

If you have resonated with the intuitive argument for the value of Direct Primary Care, you will certainly find the practical application of building your company's health benefits from the care up intriguing. There is value in considering and optimizing each component of your benefits. You can separate the decisions for how to pay for the care of your employees from choices about how to provide their health insurance.

Let's look at building on a foundation of guaranteeing your employees "free" access to value-based primary care, self-insuring a portion of potential costs beyond primary care services, and limiting exposure by purchasing stop-loss insurance. This new paradigm recognizes the reality that insurance companies, commonly referred to as the payers (in other words, they are third-party payers), don't pay for anything! Your company and your employees do.

My father had several mantras when I was growing up. One was that there are only two payers in the world: taxpayers and consumers. Can you think of any other? Employers and employees are absolutely the consumers and payers of all healthcare services. Health insurance companies are neither. They are middlemen, taking money from employers and employees to pass along to providers (after taking a healthy cut for themselves and their brokers).

The true stakeholders in healthcare are the three Ps: payers, patients, and providers. All the rest is noise and must be minimized. Your job is to look out for the interests of your employees and your company rather than the interests of your insurance broker and their employer (the BUCAH carriers). What follows is an alternative to selecting a canned BUCAH insurance option. The employer and employees may be much better off by designing benefits from the care up, which are uniquely suited to meet their needs.

## The Status Quo

There's a dance that goes on every fall all across America. Health insurance renewals are an annual ritual that involves insurance carriers adjusting (increasing) their rates and repackaging their plan offerings for brokers to present to their employer clients.

Invariably, the broker sheepishly presents the plan options from the employer's current carrier, apologizing for yet another year of shock-and-awe rate increases. They then promise to shop other carriers for better deals and play one against the other to bring rate increases down a little. If the broker can get the current carrier to come down from a 14% increase to an 11% increase in order to keep the business, they proclaim that they "saved" the employer 3%. Oh, thank you!

Of course, every plan "option" from any of the BUCAH carriers is predetermined, set in stone. The insurer alone defines the plans along with all of the details. This pick-a-card-any-card approach to fully insured group health insurance plans gives the employer a false impression that they made their own choice and are meeting the health needs of their employees to the best of their ability.

This dance always occurs close enough to the renewal date that little research or consideration of other approaches can be made, and the highest priority for the human resources personnel is to merely keep the employees happy by not rocking any boats or making significant changes. Selection of traditional fully insured medical insurance from a BUCAH carrier is a false choice for many employers and does anything but accomplish the goals of quality care and affordability for employees or employers.

Under the covers in this highly opaque system of major carrier plans are multiple misaligned incentives that all but ensure perpetual escalation of premiums and dwindling of coverage. The ACA requires insurance companies to spend 85% of the premiums they collect on medical care, or they must provide rebates to their customers. The actual cost of care must go up in order for insurance carriers to raise their rates. This medical loss ratio provision means that carriers and brokers make more money when employers spend more on insurance, when premiums go up, when employees utilize more care (and more expensive care), and when claims otherwise go up.

Neither the profits of the carrier nor the compensation of the broker is disclosed to the employer. In addition to undisclosed commissions for promoting certain plans, brokers may receive hidden bonuses and other fees to land new business or retain existing accounts, all unbeknownst to the customer.

By far, the most common BUCAH plan types are PPOs and high-deductible health plans with a savings option. A full 78% of covered employees participate in one of these two plan types. Most employers falsely assume that these plans have contracted with the highest quality doctors and healthcare systems in order to deliver better pricing and better care. PPOs are primarily designed to include as broad a network of providers as possible so they can be more attractive to employers and employees.

Most PPOs of BUCAH carriers include as many as 98% of providers available in the area and pay their providers substantially more than Medicare rates while promoting their plans as offering discounted pricing. Of course, the reality check is that those same providers routinely charge substantially lower prices to cash-paying patients without insurance than the "discounted" PPO prices.

High Deductible Health Plans (HDHP) have grown in popularity due to their lower premiums, but employees and potentially employers are assuming more risk. In the absence of guaranteed no-additional-cost access to primary care (through Direct Primary Care arrangements), high deductibles deter employees from seeking appropriate care in a timely manner, which may harm their health and result in increased costs of care in the future. Don't assume that offering a BUCAH PPO or HDHP alone will serve the needs of employees or be particularly cost effective.

This brief overview of the status quo in employer-sponsored health insurance selection and renewals illustrates that the process and products do a better job of transferring assets from employers and employees to carriers and brokers than they do in meeting the objectives for health benefits outlined in the previous chapter.

With fully insured plans, when the costs of care go up, employers and employees are sure to pay more money, and carriers and brokers are just as certain to make more. When the actual costs of care go down, BUCAH plan brokers are guaranteed to receive their (hidden) compensation and the carriers may make substantially more (undisclosed) profit. Unfortunately, employers and employees will never see a decrease in premiums or an increase in benefits as a result of containing cost.

Whoever said insanity is doing the same thing over and over and expecting different results might as well have been referring to this process. The Steve Wynn quote also applies: "The only way to win in a casino is to own one." The sooner employers recognize that their insurance carriers and brokers own the casino and have little if any incentive to improve care or save employers and employees any money, the sooner they will consider the solutions found in this book.

## Construction of Health Benefits

The paradigm that can break this dysfunctional cycle of dependence on fully insured and unnecessarily costly BUCAH plans is for you and your company to design and build each component of your health benefits to best serve the needs of your employees and your business. This means building it from the care up.

### *The Foundation of DPC*

This shift in thinking requires you to start with the foundation of providing great primary care. Hopefully by now you see the importance of guaranteed access to high-level primary care as the best way to improve employee health and patient experience and to address the drivers of healthcare costs.

This year, instead of playing pick-a-card with your current insurance agent or broker, begin by researching Direct Primary Care practices in your area. You will very likely find several. Determine if they are well established, have multiple doctors, convenient locations, excellent online reviews, and experience working with local employers.

Find out what they charge for memberships and ancillary services. DPC practices can often save employees and employers more in lab charges, expensive imaging, and prescription drugs than the entire price of their memberships. Seek references as you would for any other vendor or new hire.

Ultimately, this is the best foundation for your benefits. While you won't and shouldn't force your employees to leave their current doctor (if they have one), you are hiring the doctors that will be primarily responsible for caring for your employees and their families. The right DPC practice should also be able to guide you to benefits advisers who specialize in designing and implementing employer-directed health plans.

## *The Walls of Self-Funding*

On the foundation of Direct Primary Care, the next key building block is some form of self-insurance. Let's call this the walls. What is your company's budget for care? How much are you able to pay toward the medical care your employees need before insurance kicks in? You should be confident that your DPC doctors will engage with your employees, handle the majority of health needs within their practice, and reduce outside healthcare costs. When this starts to build over time, your company will benefit financially by directly assuming some amount of risk and cutting out the middlemen of insurance carriers and brokers.

Depending on the size of your company and your financial situation, there are several mechanisms to self-insure that should improve care and decrease cost. For the smallest companies that still wish to offer full health coverage, simply selecting a High Deductible Health Plan and then reimbursing employees for a portion of their out-of-pocket expenses until their deductible is met accomplishes the goal of partial self-funding and lowering premiums. For example, you might offer an HDHP with a $6,000 deductible, require employees to pay for the first $1,500, and then have the company pay for the remaining $4,500 thus self-insuring this portion. Of course, if most of your employees are generally healthy and utilize their DPC physician appropriately, the company will save money as few employees will have more than $1,500 in additional medical expenses in a given year.

For other companies, level-funded or fully self-funded plans may be more appropriate. Level-funding requires the employer to make set payments each month to a third-party administrator (TPA) or insurer, which funds an account that is reserved for claims, administrative costs, and premiums for stop-loss insurance (to cover any very costly claims). When claims and other costs are lower than projected, the company gets money back—something that is unheard of with BUCAH plans.

Full self-funding means that the employer is directly financially responsible for the cost of employees' medical claims. The employer contracts with a TPA or insurer to provide administrative services and typically also purchases stop-loss insurance to protect against potential very large claims.

It is crucial for employers to realize that switching to any of these types of self-insurance alone does not guarantee cost savings or better care for employees. It is only by changing the utilization habits and health habits of your employees that the triple aim of healthcare may be accomplished. Walls without the foundation of Direct Primary Care will ultimately collapse.

## *The Roof of Stop-Loss*

Very few employers will have the means to take the risk of being responsible for all medical expenses and potential catastrophic losses that could arise from their employees. They need a roof to cap their maximum exposure.

Research from the Agency for Healthcare Research and Quality indicates that 5% of the population accounts for over 50% of total healthcare spending. In most cases, even the largest employers must purchase insurance to pay for the extraordinarily large claims that may occur from a small percentage of their employees. This insurance is known as stop-loss insurance when the primary payer is a self-insured employer or reinsurance when the primary payer is an insurance plan.

In practice, HDHPs serve this function and may be considered a form of stop-loss insurance. The role of insurance is always most appropriately relegated to the function of covering only very expensive and unexpected medical expenses that an employer may not be able to afford. Leaving all of the administrative costs and profits of dealing with insurance carriers and brokers out of as much healthcare as possible and paying directly for everything you can through Direct Primary Care and self-funding should consistently improve healthcare quality, experience, and cost.

One recent alternative approach to self-insurance and stop-loss coverage that allows employers to offer insurance to their employees on the foundation of Direct Primary Care is an Individual Coverage Health Reimbursement Arrangement (ICHRA). This specific type of HRA allows employers of any size to reimburse their employees for health insurance instead of buying it for them. The ICHRA permits qualified medical expenses, including individual insurance premiums, deductibles, and copayments to be reimbursed tax-free according to design specifications and limits set by the employer.

These plans have higher limits than previous HRA and Qualified Small Employer HRA (QSEHRA) arrangements. They deliver greater choice and portability to employees and enhanced predictability of cost to the employer. An ICHRA incorporates the walls of self-funding and a known stop-loss roof for the employer without the need to directly purchase a group health insurance plan of any kind.

## *Add Doors and Windows*

To extend the analogy, there are other doors and windows features that are also important when building your health benefits from the care up. Upon the foundation of DPC, the walls of self-funding and the roof of stop-loss insurance, your company may be able to design other aspects of coverage to meet the needs of your employees and help you further manage costs in these ways:

- **Incentivize DPC Use**: You should build in incentives for employees to receive as much of their care as possible from their DPC doctor. The company can pay 100% of the costs for all services received at the DPC office including their membership fees, blood tests, imaging (x-rays, CT scans, MRI), and any other ancillary services the office may provide wholesale. All care at the DPC office is free to your employees, but they pay out-of-pocket copayments for the same services when obtained through more costly non-DPC doctors. Seeking care through DPC doctors whenever possible will save your employees money and reduce the amounts that the company will have to pay for outside medical services from its self-funded responsibility.

- **Drug Coverage**: The average American spends $115 per month on pharmaceuticals. This represents 12.6% of overall healthcare spending. Over the past few years, only 10% of prescriptions dispensed were brand-name drugs, but they are responsible for 80% of the total spent each year. When physicians prescribe medications with cost in mind and advise their patients on how to receive the lowest prices (as you should expect all DPC doctors to do), the vast majority of prescription medication needs are exceedingly cheap. Pharmacy benefits insurance is crucial for the small percentage of patients who require very expensive brand-name drugs. When building a benefit for prescription drug coverage, it is important to look for a pharmacy benefits manager (PBM) that is independent and price-transparent.

- **Provider Networks**: Your employees will sometimes need doctors other than their Direct Primary Care physician. When employees require specialty care (and for those who choose to receive care from a non-DPC primary care physician), they will want to have choices. In all cases, the employer will contract with a provider network. This network will either be determined by the carrier that is offering an HDHP or administrating self-funded options, or presented/chosen by the independent third-party administrator (TPA). In either case, the company should understand and negotiate for a favorable network with reasonable discounts whenever possible. For out-of-network coverage (and occasionally within network), the employer should consider plans that employ reference-based pricing (RBP). This payment methodology ties provider payments to a percentage of Medicare pricing rather than the more elusive "usual and customary" pricing or discounts from the typically ridiculous billed charges.

- **Direct-to-Employer Contracting**: In some cases, large employers may be able to contract directly with health systems, centers of excellence, and specialty providers to provide services with larger discounts. The healthcare providers may also assume more responsibility for the outcomes of care. These value-based arrangements that cut out the middleman create more direct accountability between the payer (employer) and the provider and allow employers to have more leverage over the costs and quality of care.
- **Prior Authorizations, Referral Management, and Step-Therapy**: Another category of plan design that can influence the efficiency and cost of care is the plan's requirement for centralized prior authorizations for procedures, referrals, and medications. These administrative hoops are designed to rein in inappropriate overutilization by providers who may have misaligned incentives or otherwise request actions that are deemed "not medically necessary" by the plan administrators. When incentives are fully aligned (as is the case with DPC providers), requirements for prior authorizations for advanced imaging tests or other diagnostics, referrals to specialists, and coverage for specific prescription medications are inefficient, do not contribute to better

care, and add a layer of unnecessary expense. They should be eliminated whenever possible.

- **Data**: Keeping score is the only way to know if you are winning or losing. If you expect to track and improve the ROI from your healthcare business, you need data. One of the biggest drawbacks to fully insured health plans is that insurance carriers do not share claims data with employers. Not only does this allow the carrier to conceal their profits, it makes it impossible for employers to identify where money is being spent and wasted or to bring about any change. They cannot "manage by fact" unless they have the facts.

  For example, if an employer had the claims data that showed they have several poorly controlled diabetics who repeatedly end up in the hospital and incur a significant percentage of the costs for the entire group, they could work on the problem. They could ask their providers to focus on the issue or contract with a diabetes center of excellence to provide specialty care that could improve the health of these few employees and bring costs down significantly. Employers who don't have all of the claims data are unable to make these kinds of quality and cost improvements.

  With any partially or fully self-funded plan, you should expect to receive detailed data. Get all of your payment data from the TPA or insurance carrier and use it to cut costs and improve care. Another source of data may be the DPC practice. While it is not always the case, your DPC physician group may be able to provide engagement data about the numbers and types of contact they have had with employees to demonstrate their active participation in the health of your workforce.

## Pick Your Builder

Your broker is your builder. You need the right builder to construct your benefits. Statistically, it is unlikely that you have selected your current health insurance broker based on how well they understand new and nontraditional approaches to health benefits and the paradigm shift recommended in this book. It's also equally unlikely that your current broker, no matter how well meaning, has a full understanding of this approach let alone meaningful experience in designing and implementing plans built on Direct Primary Care and employer-directed employee-focused self-funded plans.

If you and your company are fed up with the status quo of increasing costs, declining coverage, and poor access to care for your employees, you should consider which of these three categories your broker falls into: (1) completely qualified and experienced with designing plans as recommended in these chapters, (2) not experienced with this approach but supportive and completely willing to become educated on it and do what is in the best interest of the company, or (3) resistant to the ideas presented and not sincerely interested/willing to put effort into understanding or learning about it.

If you have a category one or two broker, they may well be the right kind of benefits adviser and not just a broker who is beholden to the major insurance carriers. If they are resistant to these concepts, you should wonder why and consider looking for an adviser who meets the criteria discussed next.

Know that DPC is a risk to brokers. DPC allows companies to buy less insurance coverage, which invariably decreases broker compensation.

What are the ideal qualities to look for in a benefits adviser? If you believe that value-based primary care delivered with the Direct Primary Care model detailed throughout this book is worth considering, you should seek an adviser who has actually worked with DPC practices and recommended/implemented plans that incorporate DPC into the plan design.

It is also important to find an adviser who understands and has experience with all types of employer self-funding. Are they able to explain in simple terms the value and mechanisms of self-funding? As discussed earlier, insurance brokers may be given incentives that do not align with those of your company or your employees. How is your broker/adviser paid? Does a significant portion of their total compensation come from the BUCAH carriers in the form of hidden commissions and kickbacks?

You should find a benefits adviser whose compensation is fully transparent. Ideally, they would be paid a simple flat fee for their work, with or without a modest success fee for how much they save your company in overall healthcare costs. Other important questions for the adviser are these:

- How do they design plans that drive the maximum number of employees to utilize DPC and how do they participate in educating your employees about changes to your health benefits?

- What relationships do they have with independent claims administrators (TPAs)? Can they obtain and share all of the claims data from the TPA and PBM to prove and manage you company's ROI?

Do you need an architect? If you have a broker/adviser that you really like, that is supportive of looking at *any* solution for your company that would be in your best interests but needs some help thinking it through from this new perspective, you may need an outside consultant to help your broker. This experienced architect can design the house, and your builder/broker can do the work of building it. There are a small handful of benefits advisers who are uniquely qualified as consultants to businesses in this situation.

If you have found a Direct Primary Care practice that you believe can meet your needs for the primary care foundation, they may be a good resource to find a consultant to perform an opportunity analysis for your company and recommend a plan design that will meet the specific needs of your business. This consultation need not threaten or displace your current benefits adviser but will lend confidence to your decision to make a (sometimes dramatic) change in how you approach health benefits. My experience is that the fee paid to the consultant/architect is well spent.

## From My Practice

At my Direct Primary Care practice in the Kansas City area, we buy what we are selling. When ProPartners Healthcare made our transition to the DPC practice model in 2013, we believed what we read and what we were told by a few DPC doctors who had gone before us. They assured us that DPC would be a win-win-win-win for patients, employers, their employees, and their doctors.

It didn't take long to verify the many ways that DPC made care more efficient and cost effective. Prior to DPC, we offered our physicians and staff a traditional BUCAH

PPO plan and watched helplessly as the premiums climbed every year, forcing us to whittle back coverage and ask our employees to contribute more (the status quo).

We made a change. As a tiny private physician-owned medical practice with about a dozen employees, we certainly couldn't be fully self-insured but believed in the concepts described about access to better care. The solution for ProPartners was to offer DPC memberships to our employees (easier for us since we are in the business) and selected an HDHP. We then self-insure the back end of the HDHP deductible. It wouldn't work without DPC as the foundation.

Our employees are responsible for the first portion of their deductible and ProPartners pays the rest. Of course, they are welcome to see other primary care physicians (paying out of their own pocket) but usually prefer to use their DPC doctor for "free." Their satisfaction with care (patient experience) is high, their out-of-pocket costs are low, and our practice has saved money on overall healthcare costs. One more example that proves breaking with the traditional approach works.

## New and Improved Approach to Health Benefits

Value-based primary care delivered through the Direct Primary Care model addresses many of the issues in the healthcare system in post-pandemic America. It is beneficial when chosen directly by individuals for their families' care and when installed by employers as the foundation of health benefits for their employees.

Companies that select their group insurance plans every year from limited BUCAH options presented by their broker have a real opportunity to make a change. Rather than selecting a plan, they can design their benefits in a way that is more likely to improve their employees' health, satisfaction with care, loyalty to their employer, and simultaneously save money for both employer and employees. Finding the right benefits adviser and consultant with experience working with DPC physicians, self-funding, and employer-directed health benefits can start your company on the road to realizing these results.

The Future of Healthcare

# Next Steps to Improve Access to Care

The value of primary care can be significant. You need a doctor who knows you and is always available to answer your questions and provide treatment right away whenever you have an issue. You need a doctor you trust. Never was that as clear as during and following the COVID-19 pandemic.

The continuity provided by an ongoing relationship with a primary care physician who delivers high-level access to care is important to your health and longevity. The value of this primary health adviser is maximized when they have the time to know their patients well, to be available whenever they are needed, and to advise patients concerning preventive care and healthy lifestyle.

Our current delivery system for primary care in America is inefficient, frustrating, and often prevents timely access to primary care doctors. A change is needed so that doctors' incentives are aligned with their patients' in a value-based practice model where non-value-added middlemen are eliminated and services are provided without individual fees for every service rendered. In other words, we need to kick the insurance companies out of the exam room.

Fortunately, membership-based Direct Primary Care (DPC) is doing just that. DPC has allowed hundreds of thousands of people from coast to coast to receive primary care more efficiently and realize the triple aim of healthcare: better care, better health, and lower costs.

DPC is not only valuable to patients who have joined DPC practices but has proven to be beneficial to forward-thinking employers who build their health benefits from the care up by installing DPC as the foundation of a plan that is designed for their unique needs.

If you have ever been frustrated by poor access to your doctor, locate Direct Primary Care physicians in your area. I can assure you they are out there. Most DPC practices are listed on the DPC Frontier website at https://mapper.dpcfrontier.com/. DPC is affordable, membership-based, insurance-free, and provides unrestricted access to primary care.

If you are an employer or decision-maker in your company and have ever been frustrated by the escalating cost of health insurance and feel helpless to do anything to buck the major medical insurance carriers' system, contact Direct Primary Care physicians in your area and make sure you have a benefits adviser who will help you design health benefits that prioritize the healthcare needs of your employees with an eye on boosting your company's bottom line too.

# End Notes

## Chapter 1

Drees, J. (2019, March 11). Google Receives More Than 1 Billion Health Questions Every Day. *Becker's Hospital Review*. Retrieved from: https://www.beckershospitalreview.com/healthcare-information-technology/google-receives-more-than-1-billion-health-questions-every-day.html#:~:text=Google's%20total%20daily%20health%2Drelated,minute%2C%20according%20to%20the%20report.

Summerton, N. (2008, April 1). The Medical History as a Diagnostic Technology. *British Journal of General Practice*, 58(549):273–276. Retrieved from: https://www.ncbi.nlm.nih.gov/pmc/articles/PMC2277113/.

## Chapter 2

CDC National Center for Health Statistics (2018). Emergency Department Visits. National Hospital Ambulatory Medical Care Survey, United States. Retrieved from: https://www.cdc.gov/nchs/fastats/emergency-department.htm.

CDC National Center for Health Statistics (2016). Accidents or Unintentional Injuries. National Ambulatory Medical Care Survey. Retrieved from: https://www.cdc.gov/nchs/fastats/accidental-injury.htm.

U.S. National Library of Medicine. Recognizing medical emergencies. Medline Plus. Retrieved from: https://medlineplus.gov/ency/article/001927.htm.

American Academy of Family Physicians (1983). Definition of Continuity of Care. American Academy of Family Physicians. Retrieved from: https://www.aafp.org/about/policies/all/continuity-of-care-definition.html.

## Chapter 3

Cruz-Cunha, M. M. (2013, April). *Handbook of Research on ICTs and Management Systems for Improving Efficiency in Healthcare and Social Care*. Retrieved from: https://www.igi-global.com/book/handbook-research-icts-management-systems/72374#table-of-contents.

Shi, L. (2012, December 31). The Impact of Primary Care: A Focused Review. *Scientifica (Cairo)*. Retrieved from: https://www.ncbi.nlm.nih.gov/pmc/articles/PMC3820521/.

Starfield, B. (2005, September). Contribution of Primary Care to Health Systems and Health. *The Milbank Quarterly*, 83(3):457–502. Retrieved from: https://www.ncbi.nlm.nih.gov/pmc/articles/PMC2690145/.

Barnett, M. (2012, January 23). Trends in Physician Referrals in the United States, 1999–2009. *Archives of Internal Medicine*, 172(2):163–170. Retrieved from: https://jamanetwork.com/journals/jamainternalmedicine/fullarticle/1108675.

Hostetter, J. (2020, July 28). Primary Care Visits Increase Utilization of Evidence-based Preventative Health Measures. *BMC Family Practice*. Retrieved from: https://bmcfampract.biomedcentral.com/articles/10.1186/s12875-020-01216-8.

Shi, L. (1992, Fall). The Relationship between Primary Care and Life Chances. *Journal of Health Care for the Poor and Underserved*. Retrieved from: https://pubmed.ncbi.nlm.nih.gov/1420668/.

Shi, L. (1994, July 1). Primary Care, Specialty Care, and Life Chances. *International Journal of Health Services*, 24(3):431–458. Retrieved from: https://pubmed.ncbi.nlm.nih.gov/7928012/.

Donohoe, M. (1998, August 10). Comparing Generalist and Specialty Care Discrepancies, Deficiencies, and Excesses. *Archives of Internal Medicine*, 158(15):1596–1608. Retrieved from: https://jamanetwork.com/journals/jamainternalmedicine/fullarticle/1105602.

Baicker, K. (2004, April 1). Medicare Spending, The Physician Workforce, and Beneficiaries' Quality of Care. *Health Affairs*. Retrieved from: https://www.healthaffairs.org/doi/abs/10.1377/hlthaff.w4.184.

## Chapter 4

Levine, D. (2020, December 16). Characteristics of Americans with Primary Care and Changes Over Time, 2002–2015. *JAMA Internal Medicine*, 180(3):463–466. Retrieved from: https://jamanetwork.com/journals/jamainternalmedicine/fullarticle/2757495.

Acklin, M. (2018, April 19). 20% of U.S. Adults Have Not Seen a Doctor in the Past Year. *Civic Science*. Retrieved from: https://civicscience.com/20-u-s-adults-not-seen-doctor-past-year/.

Borsky, A. (2018, June). Few Americans Receive All High-Priority, Appropriate Clinical Preventive Services. *Health Affairs*. Retrieved from: https://www.healthaffairs.org/doi/10.1377/hlthaff.2017.1248.

Grines, C. (2021, January 13). New Data Confirms Alarming Trend: Covid-19 Fears Are Causing Americans to Avoid the Doctor's Office and Delay Routine Care. Society for Cardiovascular Angiography and Interventions. Retrieved from: https://scai.org/new-data-confirms-alarming-trend-covid-19-fears-are-causing-americans-avoid-doctors-office-and.

Redford, G. (2020, April 27). What Makes a Good Doctor—and Other Findings from the 2019 AAMC Public Opinion Research. Association of American Medical Colleges. Retrieved from: https://www.aamc.org/news-insights/what-makes-good-doctor-and-other-findings-2019-aamc-public-opinion-research.

Miller, P. (2017). Physician Appointment Wait Times Up 30% from 2014. Merritt Hawkins. Retrieved from: https://www.merritthawkins.com/news-and-insights/media-room/press/physician-appointment-wait-times-up-from-2014/.

AANP Database (2021, May). NP Fact Sheet. American Association of Nurse Practitioners. Retrieved from: https://www.aanp.org/about/all-about-nps/np-fact-sheet.

Morton-Rias, D. (2017, March). 2016 Statistical Profile of Certified Physician Assistants. National Commission on Certification of Physician Assistants. Retrieved from: https://prodcmsstoragesa.blob.core.windows.net/uploads/files/2016StatisticalProfileofCertifiedPhysicianAssistants.pdf.

AANP (2013). Nurse Practitioners in Primary Care. American Association of Nurse Practitioners. Retrieved from: https://www.aanp.org/advocacy/advocacy-resource/position-statements/nurse-practitioners-in-primary-care.

AAMC (2020). 2020 Physician Specialty Data Report Executive Summary. Association of American Medical Colleges. Retrieved from: https://www.aamc.org/data-reports/data/2020-physician-specialty-data-report-executive-summary.

AAMC (2020, June). The Complexities of Physician Supply and Demand: Projections from 2018 to 2033. Association of American Medical Colleges. Retrieved from: https://www.aamc.org/media/45976/download.

Institute of Medicine (2008). *Retooling for an Aging America: Building the Health Care Workforce.* The National Academies Press. Retrieved from: https://www.ncbi.nlm.nih.gov/books/NBK215400/.

Sawyer, B. (2019, January 16). How Do Health Expenditures Vary across the Population? *Peterson-KFF Health System Tracker.* Retrieved from: https://www.healthsystemtracker.org/chart-collection/health-expenditures-vary-across-population/#item-people-age-55-and-over-account-for-over-half-of-total-health-spending_2016.

Hawkins, D. (2020, May 20). Primary Care Physicians Experience More Burnout and Anxiety than Other Health Professions. George Mason University College of Health and Human Services. Retrieved from: https://chhs.gmu.edu/news/2020-05/primary-care-physicians-experience-more-burnout-and-anxiety-other-health-professions.

Primary Care Collaborative. (2020, September). Quick Covid-19 Primary Care Survey—Series 21. The Larry A. Green Center and Primary Care Collaborative. Retrieved from: https://static1.squarespace.com/static/5d7ff8184cf0e01e4566cb02/t/5f75da37bde1f0691fc28b0d/1601559097041/C19+Series+21+National+Executive+Summary.pdf.

Zerehi, M. (2008, October 25). How Is a Shortage of Primary Care Physicians Affecting the Quality and Cost of Medical Care? *American College of Physicians Internal Medicine*. Retrieved from: https://www.acponline.org/acp_policy/policies/primary_care_shortage_affecting_hc_2008.pdf.

Knight, V. (2019, July 3). American Medical Students Less Likely to Choose to Become Primary Care Doctors. Kaiser Family Foundation. Retrieved from: https://khn.org/news/american-medical-students-less-likely-to-choose-to-become-primary-care-doctors/#:~:text=The%20Association%20of%20American%20Medical,whom%20have%20multiple%20chronic%20conditions.

Council on Graduate Medical Education (2010, December). Advancing Primary Care. The Council on Graduate Medical Education. Retrieved from: https://www.hopkinsmedicine.org/gim/_pdf/cogme_20_prim_care.pdf.

AAMC (2019, December). 2020 Physician Specialty Data Report: Active Physicians in the Largest Specialties, 2019. Association of American Medical Colleges. Retrieved from: https://www.aamc.org/data-reports/workforce/interactive-data/active-physicians-largest-specialties-2019.

Wilcox, L. (2021, May 26). Physician Salary Report 2021: Compensation Steady Despite COVID-19. *Weatherby Healthcare*. Retrieved from: https://weatherbyhealthcare.com/blog/annual-physician-salary-report.

Landi, H. (2019, May 7). For First Time, Employed Physicians Outnumber Self-employed Doctors, AMA Study Finds. *Fierce Healthcare*. Retrieved from: https://www.fiercehealthcare.com/practices/for-first-time-employed-physicians-outnumber-self-employed-doctors-ama-study-finds.

Merritt Hawkins (2012, September). A Survey of America's Physicians: Practice Patterns and Perspectives. The Physicians Foundation. Retrieved from: https://physiciansfoundation.org/wp-content/uploads/2017/12/Physicians_Foundation_2012_Biennial_Survey.pdf.

Merritt Hawkins (2014, September 16). Survey of 20,000 U.S. Physicians Shows 80% of Doctors Are Over-Extended or at Full Capacity. The Physicians Foundation. Retrieved from: https://physiciansfoundation.org/press-releases/survey-of-20000-u-s-physicians-shows-80-of-doctors-are-over-extended-or-at/.

Merritt Hawkins (2020, August). 2020 Survey of America's Physicians: Covid-19 Impact Edition. The Physicians Foundation. Retrieved from: https://physiciansfoundation.org/wp-content/uploads/2020/08/20-1278-Merritt-Hawkins-2020-Physicians-Foundation-Survey.6.pdf.

AHRQ (2021, June). What Is Patient Experience? Patient Experience Defined. Agency for Healthcare Research and Quality. Retrieved from: https://www.ahrq.gov/cahps/about-cahps/patient-experience/index.html.

Regina Corso Consulting (2017, October 4). The Physicians Foundation 2017 Patient Survey. The Physicians Foundation. Retrieved from: https://physiciansfoundation.org/physician-and-patient-surveys/the-physicians-foundation-2017-patient-survey/.

Consumer Reports (2013, June). What Bugs Americans Most about Their Doctors. *Consumer Reports Magazine*. Retrieved from: https://www.consumerreports.org/cro/magazine/2013/06/what-bugs-you-most-about-your-doctor/index.htm.

Raffoul, M. (2016, July 7). A Primary Care Panel Size of 2500 Is Neither Accurate nor Reasonable. *Journal of the American Board of Family Medicine*, 29(4):496–499. Retrieved from: https://www.jabfm.org/content/jabfp/29/4/496.full.pdf.

Rappleye, E. (2015, April 22). How Long Is the Average Wait at a Physician's Office? *Becker's Hospital Review*. Retrieved from: https://www.beckershospitalreview.com/hospital-physician-relationships/how-long-is-the-average-wait-at-a-physician-s-office.html.

Michas, F. (2019, August 9). Amount of Time U.S. Primary Care Physicians Spent with Each Patient as of 2018. *Statista*. Retrieved from: https://www.statista.com/statistics/250219/us-physicians-opinion-about-their-compensation/.

## Chapter 5

Merritt Hawkins (2018, September 18). The Physicians Foundation 2018 Physician Survey. The Physicians Foundation. Retrieved from: https://physiciansfoundation.org/physician-and-patient-surveys/the-physicians-foundation-2018-physician-survey/.

Thomson, K. (2021, May 10). Congress: Act Now to Ensure Telehealth Access for Medicare Beneficiaries. *Health Affairs*. Retrieved from: https://www.healthaffairs.org/do/10.1377/hblog20210505.751442/full/.

CMS (2020, March 17). Medicare Telemedicine Health Care Provider Fact Sheet. Centers for Medicare & Medicaid Services. Retrieved from: https://www.cms.gov/newsroom/fact-sheets/medicare-telemedicine-health-care-provider-fact-sheet.

Merritt Hawkins (2020, August). 2020 Survey of America's Physicians: Covid-19 Impact Edition. The Physicians Foundation. Retrieved from: https://physiciansfoundation.org/wp-content/uploads/2020/08/20-1278-Merritt-Hawkins-2020-Physicians-Foundation-Survey.6.pdf.

Basu, S. (2020, June 25). Primary Care Practice Finances in the United States Amid the COVID-19 Pandemic. *Health Affairs*. Retrieved from: https://www.healthaffairs.org/doi/full/10.1377/hlthaff.2020.00794.

Schmerker, J. (2020, May 30). Covid-19 Testing: A Brief History. *Integrated DNA Technologies*. Retrieved from: https://www.idtdna.com/pages/community/blog/post/covid-19-testing-a-brief-history.

Czeisler, M. (2020, September 11). Delay or Avoidance of Medical Care Because of COVID-19–Related Concerns—United States, June 2020. *Morbidity and Mortality Weekly Report,* 69(36):1250–1257. Retrieved from: https://www.cdc.gov/mmwr/volumes/69/wr/mm6936a4.htm.

Hamel, L. (2020, June 26). KFF Health Tracking Poll—June 2020. Kaiser Family Foundation. Retrieved from: https://www.kff.org/report-section/kff-health-tracking-poll-june-2020-social-distancing-delayed-health-care-and-a-look-ahead-to-the-2020-election/.

Panchal, N. (2021, February 10). The Implications of COVID-19 for Mental Health and Substance Use. Kaiser Family Foundation. Retrieved from: https://www.kff.org/coronavirus-covid-19/issue-brief/the-implications-of-covid-19-for-mental-health-and-substance-use/.

CDC (2020, August 20). COVID-19 Parental Resources Kit—Early Childhood: Social, Emotional, and Mental Well-being of Young Children during COVID-19. Centers for Disease Control and Prevention. Retrieved from: https://www.cdc.gov/coronavirus/2019-ncov/daily-life-coping/parental-resource-kit/early-childhood.html.

## Chapter 6

Tolbert, J. (2020, November 6). Key Facts about the Uninsured Population. Kaiser Family Foundation. Retrieved from: https://www.kff.org/uninsured/issue-brief/key-facts-about-the-uninsured-population/.

AHP (2021, March 18). A Brief History of Private Insurance in the United States. *Academic Health Plans*. Retrieved from: https://www.ahpcare.com/a-brief-history-of-private-insurance-in-the-united-states/.

BC/BS (2012, November 11). Health Insurance from Invention to Innovation: A History of the Blue Cross and Blue Shield Companies. Blue Cross Blue Shield Association. Retrieved from: https://www.bcbs.com/articles/health-insurance-invention-innovation-history-of-the-blue-cross-and-blue-shield.

Smith, G. (2021, March 5). The Complete History of Employer-Provided Health Insurance. *PeopleKeep*. Retrieved from: https://www.peoplekeep.com/blog/the-complete-history-of-employer-provided-health-insurance.

CDC (2021, July 27). Estimated COVID-19 Burden. Centers for Disease Control and Prevention. Retrieved from: https://www.cdc.gov/coronavirus/2019-ncov/cases-updates/burden.html.

HealthCare.gov (2021). Individual Coverage Health Reimbursement Arrangements (HRAs). Centers for Medicare & Medicaid. Retrieved from: https://www.healthcare.gov/small-businesses/learn-more/individual-coverage-hra/.

McCorry, D. (2014, August 6). Direct Primary Care: An Innovative Alternative to Conventional Health Insurance. The Heritage Foundation. Retrieved from: https://www.heritage.org/health-care-reform/report/direct-primary-care-innovative-alternative-conventional-health-insurance#_ftn10.

Brenan, M. (2018, December 20). Nurses Again Outpace Other Professions for Honesty, Ethics. Gallup. Retrieved from: https://news.gallup.com/poll/245597/nurses-again-outpace-professions-honesty-ethics.aspx.

Ganguli, I. (2020, February 18). Declining Use of Primary Care Among Commercially Insured Adults in the United States, 2008–2016. *Annals of Internal Medicine,* 172(4):240–247. Retrieved from: https://www.acpjournals.org/doi/10.7326/M19-1834.

CarePayment (2018, February 14). New CarePayment Research Shows Americans Can't Afford Their Medical Bills. Retrieved from: https://www.carepayment.com/new-carepayment-research-shows-americans-cant-afford-medical-bills/.

# Chapter 7

IHI (2020). The IHI Triple Aim. Institute for Healthcare Improvement. Retrieved from: http://www.ihi.org/Engage/Initiatives/TripleAim/Pages/default.aspx.

Norman, A. (2020, March 1). An Overview of the Triple Aim: A Framework to Help Healthcare Systems Optimize Performance. Verywell Health. Retrieved from: https://www.verywellhealth.com/triple-aim-4174961.

Robbins, J. (1993, January). The Influence of Physician Practice Behaviors on Patient Satisfaction. *Family Medicine,* 25(1):17–20. Retrieved from: https://pubmed.ncbi.nlm.nih.gov/8454118/.

Chandra, S. (2019, July 2). Factors Associated with Patient Satisfaction in Outpatient Department of Suva Sub-divisional Health Center, Fiji, 2018: A Mixed Method Study. *Frontiers in Public Health.* Retrieved from: https://www.ncbi.nlm.nih.gov/pmc/articles/PMC6614334/#:~:text=Studies%20have%20shown%20that%20some,trust%20(7%E2%80%9316).

HCPro (2007, April 27). The Seven Traits of Satisfied Patients. *DrScore.* Retrieved from: http://www.hcpro.com/HOM-69849-3484/The-seven-traits-of-satisfied-patients.html.

CMS (2021, March 4). Accountable Care Organizations (ACOs): What is an ACO? Centers for Medicare & Medicaid Services. Retrieved from: https://www.cms.gov/Medicare/Medicare-Fee-for-Service-Payment/ACO.

Kisling, L. (2021, May 9). *Prevention Strategies*. StatPearls Publishing. Retrieved from: https://www.ncbi.nlm.nih.gov/books/NBK537222/.

CDC (2014, July 3). Prevention: Picture of America. Centers for Disease Control & Prevention. Retrieved from: https://www.cdc.gov/pictureofamerica/pdfs/picture_of_america_prevention.pdf.

Shrank, W. (2019, October 7). Waste in the US Health Care System: Estimated Costs and Potential for Savings. *Journal of the American Medical Association*, 322(15):1501–1509. Retrieved from: https://jamanetwork.com/journals/jama/article-abstract/2752664?guestAccessKey=bf8f9802-be69-4224-a67f-42bf2c53e027&utm_source=For_The_Media&utm_medium=referral&utm_campaign=ftm_links&utm_content=tfl&utm_term=100719.

CMS (2018, February 14). CMS Office of the Actuary releases 2017–2026 Projections of National Health Expenditures. Centers for Medicare & Medicaid Services. Retrieved from: https://www.cms.gov/newsroom/press-releases/cms-office-actuary-releases-2017-2026-projections-national-health-expenditures.

Starfield, B. (2002, June). Policy Relevant Determinants of Health: An International Perspective. *Elsevier Science Health Policy*, 60(3):201–218. Retrieved from: https://www.sciencedirect.com/science/article/abs/pii/S0168851001002081.

Franks, P. (1998, August). Primary Care Physicians and Specialists as Personal Physicians. Health Care Expenditures and Mortality Experience. *Journal of Family Practice*, 47(2):105–109. Retrieved from: https://pubmed.ncbi.nlm.nih.gov/9722797/.

## Chapter 8

Treatment of Direct Primary Care Medical Home, 76 Fed. Reg. 41900 (July 15, 2011) (amending section 1301(a)(3) of the Affordable Care Act) Direct Primary Care Medical Home. Retrieved from: https://www.federalregister.gov/articles/2011/07/15/2011-17610/patient-protection-and-affordable-care-act-establishment-of-exchanges-and-qualified-health-plans

MDDI (2011, September 15). A Short History of Managed Care. *Journal of the Medical Device and Diagnostic Industry.* Retrieved from: https://www.mddionline.com/news/short-history-managed-care.

NAACOS (2021, January). Accountable Care Organizations (ACOs) Offer Enormous Opportunity for Patients and Providers. National Association of ACOs. Retrieved from: https://www.naacos.com/.

CMS (2021, July 20). Primary Care First Model Options. Centers for Medicare & Medicaid Services. Retrieved from: https://innovation.cms.gov/innovation-models/primary-care-first-model-options.

DPC Coalition (2019). What Is Direct Primary Care? Direct Primary Care Coalition. Retrieved from: https://www.dpcare.org/.

Bliss, G. (2012). Qliance Management Team. Qliance Medical Group of Washington. Retrieved from: https://qliance.com/about-us-management-team.html.

Concierge Medicine Today (2019). The History of Concierge Medicine in America (1996–Present Day). *Concierge Medicine Today*. Retrieved from: https://conciergemedicinetoday.org/the-history-of-concierge-medicine-in-america-1996-present-day/.

Eskew, P. (2021). DPC Frontier Mapper. DPC Frontier. Retrieved from: https://mapper.dpcfrontier.com/.

Bliss, G. (2011, May 12). Statement of Garrison Bliss, MD, Chief Medical Officer, Qliance Medical Group Seattle, WA: Ways and Means Subcommittee on Health Hearing on Reforming Medicare Physician Payments. Qliance Primary Care Specialists. Retrieved from: https://gop-waysandmeans.house.gov/UploadedFiles/Garrison_BlissSGR.pdf.

Qliance. (2015, January 15). New Primary Care Model Delivers 20 Percent Lower Overall Healthcare Costs, Increases Patient Satisfaction and Delivers Better Care. Qliance Medical Management. Retrieved from: https://www.prnewswire.com/news-releases/new-primary-care-model-delivers-20-percent-lower-overall-healthcare-costs-increases-patient-satisfaction-and-delivers-better-care-300021116.html.

Busch, F. (2020, May). Direct Primary Care: Evaluating a New Model of Delivery and Financing. Milliman and the Society of Actuaries. Retrieved from: https://www.soa.org/globalassets/assets/files/resources/research-report/2020/direct-primary-care-eval-model.pdf.

Chase, D. (2015, May 1). The Quadruple Aim: A Square Deal for Clinicians (& Patients). Dave Chase, LinkedIn. Retrieved from: https://www.linkedin.com/pulse/square-deal-clinicians-quadruple-aim-dave-chase/.

Bodenheimer, T. (2014, November). From Triple to Quadruple Aim: Care of the Patient Requires Care of the Provider. *Annals of Family Medicine,* 12(6):573–576. Retrieved from: https://pubmed.ncbi.nlm.nih.gov/25384822/.

Umbehr, J. (2021). Direct Primary Care Practice. Atlas MD. Retrieved from: https://atlas.md/wichita/.

Stasha, S. (2021, February 14). The State of Healthcare Industry—Statistics for 2021. *Policy Advice.* Retrieved from: https://policyadvice.net/insurance/insights/healthcare-statistics/.

## Chapter 9

Tsugawa, Y. (2018, September 26). Association between Physician US News & World Report Medical School Ranking and Patient Outcomes and Costs of Care: Observational Study. *British Medical Journal.* Retrieved from: https://www.bmj.com/content/362/bmj.k3640.

Chen, J. (2017, June 16). Relationship between Patient Satisfaction and Physician Characteristics. *Journal of Patient Experience,* 4(4):177–184. Retrieved from: https://www.ncbi.nlm.nih.gov/pmc/articles/PMC5734516/.

Jayanti, R. (2008, December 1). Like Me . . . Like Me Not: The Role of Physician Likability on Service Evaluations. *Journal of Marketing Theory and Practice,* 16(1):79–86. Retrieved from: https://www.researchgate.net/publication/247887569_Like_Me_Like_Me_Not_The_Role_of_Physician_Likability_on_Service_Evaluations.

# Chapter 10

DPC Coalition (2020). State Policy: State DPC Laws. Direct Primary Care Coalition. Retrieved from: https://www.dpcare.org/state-level-progress-and-issues.

IRS (2020, December 29). Affordable Care Act: Employer Shared Responsibility Provisions. Internal Revenue Service. Retrieved from: https://www.irs.gov/affordable-care-act/employers/employer-shared-responsibility-provisions.

KFF (2019). State Health Facts: Health Insurance Coverage of the Total Population. Kaiser Family Foundation. Retrieved from: https://www.kff.org/other/state-indicator/total-population/?currentTimeframe=0&sortModel=%7B%22colId%22:%22Location%22,%22sort%22:%22asc%22%7D.

KFF (2020, October 8). 2020 Employer Health Benefits Survey. Kaiser Family Foundation. Retrieved from: https://www.kff.org/report-section/ehbs-2020-summary-of-findings/.

Norris, L. (2021, March 11). Will You Receive an ACA Premium Subsidy? How the Affordable Care Act's Subsidies Are Calculated, and Who Is Eligible to Receive Them under the American Rescue Plan. *IHC Specialty Benefits*. Retrieved from: https://www.healthinsurance.org/obamacare/will-you-receive-an-aca-premium-subsidy/.

HealthCare.gov (2021). High Deductible Health Plan (HDHP). Centers for Medicare & Medicaid Services. Retrieved from: https://www.healthcare.gov/glossary/high-deductible-health-plan/.

IRS (2021, January 8). Publication 502: Medical and Dental Expenses (Including the Health Coverage Tax Credit). Internal Revenue Service. Retrieved from: https://www.irs.gov/pub/irs-pdf/p502.pdf.

IRS (2019, June 20). Health Reimbursement Arrangements and Other Account-Based Group Health Plans. *Federal Register: Internal Revenue Service*. Retrieved from: https://www.govinfo.gov/content/pkg/FR-2019-06-20/pdf/2019-12571.pdf.

HealthCare.gov (2021). Flexible Spending Account (FSA). Centers for Medicare & Medicaid Services. Retrieved from: https://www.healthcare.gov/glossary/flexible-spending-account-fsa/.

Cassidy, B. (2021, January 28). S.128—Primary Care Enhancement Act of 2021. 117th Congress (2021–2022). Retrieved from: https://www.congress.gov/bill/117th-congress/senate-bill/128/text.

KFF (2019). State Health Facts: Health Insurance Coverage of the Total Population. Kaiser Family Foundation. Retrieved from: https://www.kff.org/other/state-indicator/total-population/?currentTimeframe=0&sortModel=%7B%22colId%22:%22Location%22,%22sort%22:%22asc%22%7D.

Hamel, L. (2016, May 20). Survey of Non-Group Health Insurance Enrollees, Wave 3. Kaiser Family Foundation. Retrieved from: https://www.kff.org/health-reform/poll-finding/survey-of-non-group-health-insurance-enrollees-wave-3/.

Loftsgordon, A. (2021). Obamacare: Health Insurance Marketplace Overview. *NOLO*. Retrieved from: https://www.nolo.com/legal-encyclopedia/health-insurance-marketplace-overview.html.

CMS (2021, June 2). State-based Exchanges. Centers for Medicare & Medicaid Services. Retrieved from: https://www.cms.gov/CCIIO/Resources/Fact-Sheets-and-FAQs/state-marketplaces.

HealthCare.gov (2015, May 1). People with Coverage through a Job: If You'd Like to Change to a Marketplace Plan. Centers for Medicare & Medicaid. Retrieved from: https://www.healthcare.gov/have-job-based-coverage/change-to-marketplace-plan/.

Ballotpedia (2017). Obamacare Exchange Enrollment and Subsidies by State. *Ballotpedia*. Retrieved from: https://ballotpedia.org/Obamacare_exchange_enrollment_and_subsidies_by_state.

HealthCare.gov (2021). New, Lower Costs on Marketplace Coverage. Centers for Medicare & Medicaid. Retrieved from: https://www.healthcare.gov/more-savings/.

Kamal, R. (2018, October 26). How Repeal of the Individual Mandate and Expansion of Loosely Regulated Plans Are Affecting 2019 Premiums. Kaiser Family Foundation. Retrieved from: https://www.kff.org/health-costs/issue-brief/how-repeal-of-the-individual-mandate-and-expansion-of-loosely-regulated-plans-are-affecting-2019-premiums/.

Norris, L. (2021, March 29). What Happens If I Don't Buy ACA-Compliant Health Insurance? *IHC Specialty Benefits*. Retrieved from: https://www.healthinsurance.org/faqs/what-happens-if-i-dont-buy-aca-compliant-health-insurance/.

AHCSM (2021). By the Numbers: Data and Statistics. Alliance of Health Care Sharing Ministries. Retrieved from: http://ahcsm.org/about-us/data-and-statistics/.

## Chapter 11

HealthCare.gov (2021). The Small Business Health Care Tax Credit. Centers for Medicare & Medicaid. Retrieved from: https://www.healthcare.gov/small-businesses/provide-shop-coverage/small-business-tax-credits/.

TCHS (2019, October 15). Americans Largely Pleased with Health Coverage but Concerned about Affordability: New Survey Finds More Than Half of Workers Stay at Their Job to Keep Health Benefits. Transamerica Center for Health Studies. Retrieved from: https://www.prnewswire.com/news-releases/americans-largely-pleased-with-health-coverage-but-concerned-about-affordability-300938282.html.

EBRI (2018, April 26). EBRI Finds a Strong Link between Benefits Satisfaction and Job Satisfaction. Employee Benefit Research Institute. Retrieved from: https://www.ebri.org/docs/default-source/ebri-press-release/pr-1211-1-wbs-26apr18.pdf?sfvrsn=6d3a342f_4.

CDC (2015, December 4). Increase Productivity: Workplace Health Programs Can Increase Productivity. Centers for Disease Control and Prevention. Retrieved from: https://www.cdc.gov/workplacehealthpromotion/model/control-costs/benefits/productivity.html.

Stone, M. (2003, June 14). What Patients Want from Their Doctors. *British Medical Journal,* 326(7402):1294. Retrieved from: https://www.ncbi.nlm.nih.gov/pmc/articles/PMC1126182/.

Chase, D. (2017, September 4). *CEO's Guide to Restoring the American Dream: How to Deliver World Class Healthcare to Your Employees at Half the Cost.* Health Rosetta Publications. Retrieved from: https://healthrosetta.org/ceoguide/.

PGPF (2019, May 1). Healthcare Costs for Americans Projected to Grow at an Alarmingly High Rate. Peter G. Peterson Foundation. Retrieved from: https://www.pgpf.org/blog/2019/05/healthcare-costs-for-americans-projected-to-grow-at-an-alarmingly-high-rate.

Callahan, D. (2015, September 23). Health Care Costs and Medical Technology. The Hastings Center. Retrieved from: https://www.thehastingscenter.org/briefingbook/health-care-costs-and-medical-technology/.

CMS (2020, December 16). CMS Office of the Actuary Releases 2019 National Health Expenditures. Centers for Medicare & Medicaid Services. Retrieved from: https://www.cms.gov/newsroom/press-releases/cms-office-actuary-releases-2019-national-health-expenditures#:~:text=Retail%20prescription%20drug%20spending%20(10,growth%20of%203.8%25%20in%202018.

Accenture (2021, June 2). Fraud, Waste and Abuse in Social Services: Identifying and Overcoming This Modern-Day Epidemic. Accenture. Retrieved from: https://www.accenture.com/be-en/insight-fraud-waste-abuse-social-services-summary.

Himmelstein, D. (2020, January 21). Health Care Administrative Costs in the United States and Canada, 2017. *Annals of Internal Medicine,* 172:134–142. Retrieved from: https://www.acpjournals.org/doi/10.7326/M19-2818?stream=top&utm_campaign=newsletter_axiosvitals&utm_medium=email&utm_source=newsletter.

Ezzati, M. (2009, April 28). Smoking, High Blood Pressure and Being Overweight Top Three Preventable Causes of Death in the U.S. Harvard School of Public Health. Retrieved from: https://web.archive.org/web/20121122110650/http:/www.hsph.harvard.edu/news/press-releases/2009-releases/smoking-high-blood-pressure-overweight-preventable-causes-death-us.html.

CDC (2014, May 1). Up to 40 percent of annual deaths from each of five leading US causes are preventable. Centers for Disease Control and Prevention. Retrieved from: https://www.cdc.gov/media/releases/2014/p0501-preventable-deaths.html.

Galea, S. (2020, October). The Cost of Preventable Disease in the USA. *The Lancet Public Health.* Retrieved from: https://www.thelancet.com/journals/lanpub/article/PIIS2468-2667(20)30204-8/fulltext.

Kakushadze, Z. (2017, September 4). Estimating Cost Savings from Early Cancer Diagnosis. *MDPI.* Retrieved from: https://www.mdpi.com/2306-5729/2/3/30/htm.

United Health Group (2019, July). 18 Million Avoidable Hospital Emergency Department Visits Add $32 Billion in Costs to the Health Care System Each Year. United Health Group. Retrieved from: https://www.unitedhealthgroup.com/content/dam/UHG/PDF/2019/UHG-Avoidable-ED-Visits.pdf.

Van Nuys, K. (2018, March 12). Overpaying for Prescription Drugs: The Copay Clawback Phenomenon. USC Leonard D. Schaeffer Center for Health Policy & Economics. Retrieved from: https://healthpolicy.usc.edu/research/overpaying-for-prescription-drugs/.

## Chapter 12

Price, S. (2021, May 24). Largest Health Insurance Companies of 2021. ValuePenguin. Retrieved from: https://www.valuepenguin.com/largest-health-insurance-companies.

KFF (2020, October 8). 2020 Employer Health Benefits Survey. Kaiser Family Foundation. Retrieved from: https://www.kff.org/report-section/ehbs-2020-summary-of-findings/.

CMS (2020). Health Insurance Market Reforms: Medical Loss Ratio. Centers for Medicare & Medicaid Services. Retrieved from: https://www.cms.gov/CCIIO/Programs-and-Initiatives/Health-Insurance-Market-Reforms/Medical-Loss-Ratio#:~:text=The%20Affordable%20Care%20Act%20requires%20insurance%20companies%20to%20spend%20at,on%20health%20insurance%20rate%20increases.

KFF (2020, October 8). 2020 Employer Health Benefits Survey. Kaiser Family Foundation. Retrieved from: https://www.kff.org/report-section/ehbs-2020-summary-of-findings/.

Mitchell, E. (2020, February). Concentration of Healthcare Expenditures and Selected Characteristics of High Spenders, U.S. Civilian Noninstitutionalized Population, 2017. Agency for Healthcare Research and Quality. Retrieved from: https://meps.ahrq.gov/data_files/publications/st528/stat528.shtml.

OECD (2019, November 7). Health at a Glance 2019: Pharmaceutical Spending. Organisation for Economic Co-operation and Development. Retrieved from: https://data.oecd.org/healthres/pharmaceutical-spending.htm.

Mikulic, M. (2020, August 18). Branded vs. Generic U.S. Drug Prescriptions Dispensed 2005–2019. *Statista*. Retrieved from: https://www.statista.com/statistics/205042/proportion-of-brand-to-generic-prescriptions-dispensed/.

Mikulic, M. (2020, August 18). Proportion of Branded versus Generic Prescription Drug Revenues in the United States from 2005 to 2019. *Statista*. Retrieved from: https://www.statista.com/statistics/205036/proportion-of-brand-to-generic-prescription-sales/.

Phia Group (2021). Reference-Based Pricing Explained. The Phia Group. Retrieved from: https://www.phiagroup.com/Media/Referenced-Based-Pricing-Explained.

Gaal, M. (2019, July 19). Is Direct-to-Provider Contracting a Potential Silver Bullet for Achieving Value-based Care for Employer-sponsored Plans? Milliman. Retrieved from: https://www.milliman.com/en/insight/is-direct-to-provider-contracting-a-potential-silver-bullet-for-achieving-value-based-care.

# Acknowledgments

The grass of primary care is becoming greener across America due to a couple thousand roots that have taken hold. Thank you to the grassroots, the Direct Primary Care (DPC) physicians who have risked their traditional employment and insurance-based careers to pioneer a better, faster, and cheaper model for delivering frontline healthcare over the past twenty-five years. You have sparked a compassionate revolution.

To all the organizations and individuals who have encouraged the growth of the DPC movement, whether we have met or I have watched and learned from you from afar, I want to thank you for your commitment to supporting, encouraging, and inspiring all of the DPC doctors, myself included, to pursue and succeed at the vision of direct value-based care.

I would also like to thank the more than 2,000 patients of ProPartners Healthcare, PA, who were willing to see outside of the participating provider box, become members of a different kind of primary care practice, and pay their doctor to simply be available. It has been an honor to know you and care for you as a proactive partner in your health.

Without the commitment and support of the physicians and staff at ProPartners Healthcare over the past twenty years, this book would not exist. Every one of you has proven the contents of this book to be true in the real world of primary care. You have allowed me to confidently extol the value of DPC from countless examples of care delivered with excellence, timeliness, and great compassion. I'm extremely grateful to Sonny, Angela, Vonda, Martha, Becky, Kristi, Jannah, Heide, Cheri, Sonya, Amy, Shari, and many past team members.

I didn't intend to write a book. My fifteen-page white paper kind of morphed into everything I had to say about primary care. Since they didn't teach me to write in medical school, I was desperate for help and am extremely grateful to have found an experienced and insightful editor, Sandra Wendel. Many thanks to Sandra, Craig Scurato, Dan Meylan, Jay Keese, Nicholas Comninellis, Scott Stevens, Vonda Accurso, Alexander von Ness, and Megan McCullough who focused and scrubbed the material, designed a professional look, kept me from embarrassing myself, and helped make this book happen.

I had never heard of Direct Primary Care until my partners, Charles "Sonny" Holbrook, III, MD, and Clark Eddy, DO, introduced me to the idea in 2013. I was not only skeptical but quite resistant. They saw the future, the many benefits of DPC and how it could apply to our practice. I didn't. The risks of "firing" our 9,000 patients and their insurance carriers seemed too high. Eight years later, I can say it was the best business and personal decision we could have made. I am deeply indebted to Sonny for his insight, investment in ProPartners, and faithfulness to the vision and to me personally over the past sixteen years.

Special thanks to my adult children (four biologicals and two sons-in-law): Amy, Tim, Jenna, Kevin, Chris, and

Kari. You have each changed my life for the better and have provided countless opportunities for me to work on caring, communication skills, and teaching over the past thirty years. You will have to decide if those opportunities have made me a better father but they have certainly made me a better doctor. I am "sinfully proud" of each of you.

Finally, to my wonderful wife and best friend, Cathy, I am forever blessed with your unwavering love and support in the midst of the thirty-three years that you have indulged my entrepreneurial bent. You have been my partner and hung on for the ride in starting and building multiple businesses, churches, schools, bands, homes, and the most amazing of all families. Of all your wonderful and widely recognized qualities, I am amazed by your love for me the most. I love you.

# About the Author

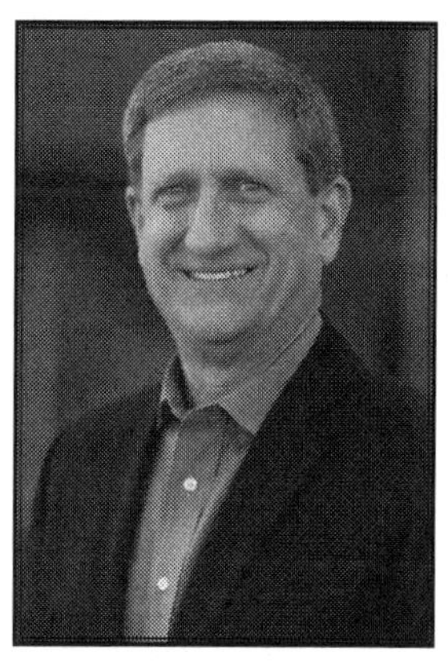

**Troy A. Burns, MD,** is a practicing primary care physician and the Founder and Medical Director of ProPartners Healthcare, Kansas City's leading Direct Primary Care medical practice. He also serves on the Steering Committee of the Direct Primary Care Coalition, an advocacy group in Washington, DC, which represents physicians, healthcare associations, employers, and others who support the advancement of policies that promote better primary care.

Dr. Burns previously founded and built a multistate medical practice specializing in men's health with thirty-six practices in twenty-three states. He received his medical degree from the University of Missouri at Kansas City in 1986 and completed an Internal Medicine internship at St. Luke's Hospital in Kansas City.

Dr. Burns is a husband, father of four, father-in-law of two and "gramps" of two. He is a vocalist and keyboardist, having played for decades in classic rock bands and on church worship teams. He and his wife, Cathy, also teach parenting classes through their local church.

Visit Dr. Burns online at www.propartnershealthcare.com.

Made in the USA
Columbia, SC
01 December 2021

50173590R00133